DATE DUE

NOV 20 2000	
NOV 21 2001	
Dec. 4, 2001	
MAY 4 2002	
MAY 7 2002	
MAR 29 2004	

ETHICAL ISSUES IN HIV VACCINE TRIALS

Ethical Issues in HIV Vaccine Trials

Thomas A. Kerns
North Seattle Community College
Seattle, Washington

First published in Great Britain 1997 by
MACMILLAN PRESS LTD
Houndmills, Basingstoke, Hampshire RG21 6XS and London
Companies and representatives throughout the world

A catalogue record for this book is available from the British Library.

ISBN 0–333–66597–X hardcover
ISBN 0–333–67492–8 paperback

First published in the United States of America 1997 by
ST. MARTIN'S PRESS, INC.,
Scholarly and Reference Division,
175 Fifth Avenue, New York, N.Y. 10010

ISBN 0–312–16397–5

Library of Congress Cataloging-in-Publication Data
Kerns, Thomas A., 1942–
Ethical issues in HIV vaccine trials / Thomas A. Kerns.
p. cm.
Includes bibliographical references and index.
ISBN 0–312–16397–5 (cloth)
1. AIDS vaccines—Research—Moral and ethical aspects—Developing countries. 2. Human experimentation in medicine—Moral and ethical aspects—Developing countries. I. Title.
QR189.5.A33K47 1996
174'.28—dc20 96–25611
CIP

---

10 9 8 7 6 5 4 3 2 1
06 05 04 03 02 01 00 99 98 97

Printed and bound in Great Britain by
Antony Rowe Ltd, Chippenham, Wiltshire

Contents

Dedication

To Mother, Tops Manglesdorf Kerns RN, mother of all mothers, a soul who laughs and brings fun into the world, even in the morning, even raising eight kids; staunch protector and defender of her chicks, bringer of cheerfulness into a world desperately in need of it.

To Dad, T. A. Kerns, MD, father extraordinaire, dear and glorious physician, healer of souls, man of wisdom, life teacher of his children, spiritual exemplar, founder of schools, founder of treatment centers, devout follower of his God.

Two of the greatest souls I've known, and whom I love beyond measure. Everyone who knows them loves and cherishes them. I count it the greatest privilege to have been born to them, and to be the brother of the seven best and funnest siblings in the world, Janie, Patsy, Bob, Mary K., Bwill, John and Pete.

To Mother and Dad I dedicate this book, as one more small expression of a limitless love and gratitude.

AIDS is the single greatest threat to well-being facing the world's population today.

Marc Lappé[1]

One legacy of the "miracle drugs," the antibiotics of the 1940s, has been an extraordinary complacency on the part of the broader culture. Most people today are grossly overoptimistic with respect to the means we have available to forfend global epidemics comparable to the Black Death of the fourteenth century (or, on a lesser scale, the influenza of 1918), which took a toll of millions of lives! We have no guarantee that the natural evolutionary competition of viruses with the human species will always find ourselves the winner.

Joshua Lederberg[2]

I am a member of a fragile species, still new to the earth, the youngest creatures of any scale, here only a few moments as evolutionary time is measured, a juvenile species, a child of a species. We are only tentatively set in place, error-prone, at risk of fumbling, in real danger at the moment of leaving behind only a thin layer of our fossils, radioactive at that.

Lewis Thomas[3]

Scientists should continue to do research. But if a human being is ever used in the experiments, the scientists must make a moral commitment never to violate a person's human rights and human dignity. Every time scientists are involved in human experimentation, they should try to put themselves in the place of the subject and see how they would feel.

Mrs Eva Mozes-Kor

So act as to treat humanity, whether in thine own person or in that of any other, in every case as an end withal, never as a means only.

Immanuel Kant[4]

When spiders unite, they can tie up a lion.

Ethiopian proverb

No man is an island, entire of itself; every man is a piece of the continent, a part of the main. If a clod be washed away by the sea, Europe is the less, as well as if a promontory were. . . . Any man's death diminishes me because I am involved in mankind, and therefore never send to know for whom the bell tolls; it tolls for thee.

John Donne

A little learning is a dangerous thing; drink deep or taste not the Pierian Spring.

Alexander Pope

NOTES

1. M. Lappé. *Evolutionary Medicine: Rethinking the Origins of Disease* (San Francisco, CA: Sierra Club Books, 1994) 255+xii, p 109.
2. A. Mack, ed. *In Time of Plague: The History and Social Consequences of Lethal Epidemic Disease* (New York: New York University Press, 1991) 206+xii., p 24.
3. L. Thomas. *The Fragile Species* (New York, NY: Charles Scribner's Sons, 1992) 193+xii., p 25.
4. I. Kant. *Fundamental Principles of the Metaphysic of Morals,* Trans. Thomas Kingsmill Abbott. vol 42 of 54, (Chicago, IL: *The Great Books of the Western World, Encyclopedia Britannica,* Inc, 1785, 1952), p 272.

Preface

Difficult as it may be for us to acknowledge, a fulminant epidemic is already well upon us.

That which is already upon us, of course, can no longer be prevented (if it ever could have been). What might still be preventable, however, is the increasingly dramatic acceleration of the AIDS pandemic around the globe. This book is about the ethical issues facing those who are struggling to control, with a vaccine, a pandemic that gives every impression of being already out of control.

Ancient Greek tradition honored the medical art of healing, under the form of the god Aesklepios, and honored the medical art of prevention, under the form of the goddess Hygeia. No one who has ever been healed from a sickness will want to minimize the importance of the art of healing as performed by a skilled and caring physician. Equally important, however, is the medical art of prevention. The small statue of the goddess Hygeia, which stands just outside the main entrance to the World Health Organization in Geneva, symbolizes that organization's commitment to the prevention of sickness and suffering.

This book too reflects the goddess more than the god. It is about prevention.

It is about minimizing suffering and maximizing hope and well-being in a struggling and imperfect world.

It is about protecting the rights and well-being of human beings who themselves are imperfect, who suffer, who are flawed, yet who live hope-filled lives.

This is a book about a complex, difficult, and extremely important question. The question is this: How, when, where, under what conditions, and on whom shall we test experimental AIDS vaccines?

As an academic, I have been blessed with the freedom to reflect on these matters without any built-in bias: I neither work for, nor have a financial interest in, any pharmaceutical company or medical establishment. I am not part of any government or agency that is promoting vaccine trials. I have no financial interest in wanting candidate vaccines to get tested. Nor have I any special interest, financial or otherwise, in wanting candidate vaccines to not get tested. I do, in fact, still have a rather warm hope that some form of a moderately successful AIDS vaccine will eventually be developed.

If it ever turns out to be the case that there are persons with a naturally occurring immunity to HIV infection and AIDS (as, for example, the long-term survivors, or the long-term non-progressors, or the Gambian commercial sex workers in recent news stories,[5] or any of the individuals with apparent immunities to HIV periodically reported in the press), then that will indeed be a significant ray of hope for those searching for a vaccine.

In any case, this book is not an argument for or against the testing of HIV vaccines, except in so far as such vaccines could be part of a successful strategy for slowing or stopping the pandemic.

Nor is this book an argument for one side or the other of most of the ethical questions it raises (although it does take a position on some of the central questions raised in the Introduction).

What this book is trying to be, rather, is an exploration of, and a journey through, some of the central ethical issues that need to be discussed prior to undertaking large scale human efficacy trials, either in the industrialized world or in developing nations.

The purpose of this book, then, to say it in the simplest terms, is to pose the questions, to lay them out in all their stark plainness, and in all their troublesome complexity. It will lie with another, later book to propose answers to some of these dilemmas. This book is primarily an attempt to articulate and clarify the questions, questions which will, I hope, stimulate large scale public discussion. This purpose arises from a deeply held belief that it is only in the clear posing of good questions that any adequate answers will ever be discovered.

AIDS vaccine research is of crucial human importance, whether it ultimately proves to be fruitful or not. It is a drama that fully deserves its hour on center stage. Although one author believes that "the eyes of the world are on HIV vaccine researchers, today more than ever,"[6] I believe that the spotlights on HIV vaccine research will not reach their fullest focus for another two or three years. This research is exceptionally important, and very much deserves our attention and our scrutiny. It deserves our very best thinking.

This book intends to raise the issues, to explore their various sides, and to encourage public discourse about the crucially important global policy questions entailed by this research.

In the arena of HIV and AIDS there are, of course, a wide variety of very complex, powerful, and controversial ethical issues. In my regular teaching of a Medical Ethics course which is devoted exclusively to ethical and policy issues related to HIV and AIDS, we explore as many of those issues as we can fit into one college term. This book, however, focuses on only a very small subset of those ethical problems, namely, the ethical issues concerned with testing HIV vaccines in persons who are *not* infected with HIV.

One final prefatory note: the existentialist philosopher Soren Kierkegaard has one of his pseudonymous authors (Johannes Climacus) ironically note that all the famous authors of his day seem to want to "make spiritual existence . . . easier and easier" for people. Climacus concludes that the only thing left for him to do is to make things harder and harder for people. "I conceived it as my task [he says] to create difficulties everywhere."[7]

Unlike Kierkegaard's ironical pseudonym, I do not conceive it as my task to create difficulties everywhere. I do, however, conceive it as one task of this book to recognize, to acknowledge, and to make known the wide and varied array of ethical difficulties that do already exist in the prospect of designing these trials. I hope that creative minds will find ways to design these trials so that we can deal fairly and justly with the persons who decide to volunteer for them, and so we can make the trials successful in answering the scientific questions posed to them.

NOTES

5. S. Rowland-Jones, "HIV-specific Cytotoxic T-cells in HIV-exposed but Uninfected Gambian Women", *Nature Medicine*, 1 January (1995) 59–64. See also: Associated Press. "Gambian group have rare immunity to AIDS virus." *The Seattle Times* 1 January 1995.
6. Associated Press "Researchers Look to Girl, 13, for Clues on AIDS." *The New York Times* 9 January 1995. A10., 314.
7. S. Kierkegaard and J. (Climacus. Kierkegaard's Concluding Unscientific Postscript. Trans. Swenson, David and Lowrie, Walter, Princeton University Press, 1846, 1941) 577+xxii., p 166.

Acknowledgements

With immense gratitude . . .

- for careful reading with copious comments: to Renee, my daughter Lisa, my brother Bob, students in philosophy 100, and friends and colleagues, especially Bill Reed, Jim Harnish, Andrea Wyatt, Gail Baker, and Fran Schmitt;
- for encouragement, research help, answers to questions, and for numerous suggestions: to Drs José Esparza, William Heyward, and Peter Piot of UNAIDS:
- for encouragement and support: to Renee, Lisa, Bill Reed, Kate Lindemann, and for strong support encouragement and belief in the project, Dad and Mother; and all my brothers and sisters (particularly Brother Peter, who said, "It sure doesn't take a rocket scientist to understand this stuff, does it?");
- for financial assistance: to Bruce Kochis and the NSCC International Studies Program; The University of Washington/Bothell Conference on Human Rights; and North Seattle Community College, for a sabbatical and some small travel grants;
- for help keeping me sane, and reminding me of what's truly important: to all my siblings, my son Tom, daughters Lisa and Roxanne, and friend and running partner Neil Clough.

Most of what is valuable or useful in this book is due to their generosity; responsibility for the errors is mine alone.

Introduction

Ethical predicaments emerge from every quarter when we try to test HIV vaccines in human subjects.

Moreover, the ethical complexities multiply like the Hydra's head, and become even more challenging when the populations in which we want to test these vaccines are among the more disadvantaged, poor and oppressed peoples of the earth.

The purpose of this book is to lay out the details of these ethical questions so they can become part of the public discourse. These trials, already in the planning and initial implementation stages, raise ethical difficulties at least as complex as (perhaps more complex than) any ethical problems we have yet had to deal with in human subjects research.[1] Policymakers can expect to be faced with some extremely difficult choices in the years just ahead.

In a hotly debated decision in June of 1994, the United States National Institutes of Health chose to reject the application for large scale HIV vaccine efficacy trials with the gp120 candidate vaccines developed by Genentech and Biocene. The reasons, though never fully articulated, may have included some of the following. Perhaps it was believed there was too little chance that the vaccines would prove successful. Or perhaps it was believed that expensive efficacy trials were not the best way to allocate scarce AIDS resources. Or perhaps there was simply too much political pressure from AIDS activists. Or perhaps it was one of a host of other possible reasons, varying according to your place among the meeting's constituencies.[2]

Then, in October of 1994, four months later, a consultative meeting of AIDS experts from around the globe convened at the World Health Organization's Global Programme on AIDS in Geneva to address the same question: whether or not to recommend large scale efficacy trials for the same type of candidate vaccine. This group heard testimony, deliberated, discussed and finally concluded that large scale efficacy trials could be conducted (subject to the initiative and final decision of the host country) in one (or more) of three developing nations:

> The World Health Organization announced Friday that it had approved the first large-scale trials of possible HIV vaccines. The unnamed vaccines will be tested in Brazil, Uganda, and [Thailand]. The announcement came after a two-day meeting in Geneva, in which experts agreed that some genetically-engineered vaccines had proven in preliminary trials to be safe and to help create HIV immunity.[3]

This juxtaposition of these two opposite judgments by two reflective and responsible world organizations should alert us to the fact that the questions they are dealing with are extremely controversial. The questions are controversial because the science involved is complex, difficult, and rich with ambiguities; because the politics involved is so multifaceted; and because the ethical issues involved are so complicated, difficult and open to varied interpretations. Though this book will look briefly at some of the science and politics involved, it will focus primarily on the ethical issues raised by the prospect of undertaking these trials.

The clearest way to lay out the complexity of these ethical quandaries is to formulate them in terms of the two primary opposing[4] positions, one of which will be termed the Thesis position, and the other of which will be termed the Antithesis position. The central effort of this book, then, will be to articulate the thinking of each of these two positions as clearly as possible, in hopes that a fuller, more informed discussion of each will eventually yield (if Hegel can be trusted) a viable Synthesis position.

The *Thesis* statement will be articulated thus:

> In the face of so much growing personal tragedy associated with HIV infection, and in the face of such a rapidly expanding global pandemic, waiting any longer to initiate phase I and II trials for HIV vaccines is simply wrong. These trials must be initiated immediately, so that we can

quickly move on to large scale efficacy trials as soon as it is scientifically, politically, and ethically feasible.

The opposing *Antithesis* statement will be phrased thus:

> We must, under no circumstances, begin phase I, II, or III HIV vaccine trials until we can insure that the individual rights and well-being of all those who volunteer for the trials will be protected to the fullest extent possible, as required by *The Nuremberg Code* and the WHO/CIOMS *International Ethical Guidelines for Biomedical Research Involving Human Subjects.* Anything short of full compliance with these guidelines would be wrong, would be a violation of internationally accepted ethical codes, and would endanger any potential successful outcome of these trials; it may even have disastrous consequences that would impact future research protocols (as the legacy of the Tuskegee study haunts the efforts of medical researchers still today).

Each of these positions represents a strong moral stance, and each position, as we will see, defends its stance with clearly articulated reasons.

Though the US and WHO meetings were considering two quite different epidemic situations, the position taken by the US NIH as a result of its June 1994 meeting is more reflective of the sentiments expressed by the Antithesis position, and the position taken by the WHO/GPA consultative group in October of 1994 is more reflective of the sentiments expressed by the Thesis position.

The focus of this book will be to deal most fully with the ethical issues entailed by the Antithesis position. The reasons for holding the Thesis position, however, are quite compelling and deserve to be stated clearly. They are, in fact, so strong as to almost demand assent. They will include the following arguments.

We must initiate large scale efficacy trials for HIV preventive vaccines as soon as politically and ethically feasible, says the Thesis position, because:

1 The epidemic is daily growing worse; indeed it is accelerating. It is no exaggeration to say that the global HIV/AIDS pandemic is out of control.

2 Because of the high incidence of new HIV infections, the viral pool is increasing daily. This daily increase in the viral pool leads to two serious consequences:
   a As the pool of viral particles grows, the opportunities for new infections also increase. The larger the viral pool, the higher the incidence of new infections; i.e., the faster it grows, the faster it grows.
   b As the viral pool increases, the chances for new and more pathogenic variants of HIV to develop also increases. In theory, at least, there is nothing to prevent the emergence of new variants that are more readily transmissible (Joshua Lederberg has raised the possibility even of airborne variants of HIV), or variants that cause faster progression to disease, or cause worse disease (if that is possible), or the emergence of variants that are even more readily resistant to the few treatments we have available.

3 The immense burden of personal tragedy is also increasing daily. Every day that we do not have a vaccine, every day that we delay testing of candidate vaccines, is another quantum increase of approximately 10,000 (in 1995)[5] new individual infections and new personal tragedies.

4 The economic impact, particularly in developing communities, is already serious and is growing daily more severe. These costs are already devastating in some communities, as we will see, and are expected to become even more dramatic.

   When measured in years of potential life lost (YPLL), the impact of the pandemic is particularly severe because the age group that is most susceptible to infection is so young. It is also the age group, of course, that does much of the productive work in a society, and that does most of the child care in families as well.

5 The mutual interactions between HIV disease and tuberculosis have contributed to an increasingly severe recrudescence of TB (which is the one opportunistic infection that can be readily transmitted to non-HIV-infected persons), and to increasingly numerous strains of multi-drug-resistant TB (MDRTB). These developing TB epidemics around the world also take their own tolls on persons, on families, and on regional economies.

6 Nor can we ignore the possibility of HIV's developing interactions with other microbes in a manner that could potentiate either or both of them. Although there is as yet no evidence for this in present strains of HIV, the longer we wait before gaining control of the AIDS pandemic, the greater potential there is for unanticipated interactions to develop between HIV and other microbes.

7 Finally, must we not acknowledge that when the well-being of the larger community is at risk, it may be best that certain forms of individual freedom be temporarily modified. The concepts of legal military conscription, of laws of taxation, of regional zoning ordinances, and so on, are all based on the principle that sometimes individual freedoms must be temporarily modified for the well-being of the larger community. In the case of the HIV/AIDS pandemic, some societies (and even the larger human community) seem to be at significant risk. If it is even partially true that "AIDS is the single greatest threat to well-being facing the world's population today,"[6] then, in order to develop a successful preventive measure such as a vaccine, some codes and guidelines that have usually governed medical research in the developed world may need to temporarily take a back seat to the needs of the larger community, until we find some ways to get this pandemic under adequate control.

All these reasons provide strong support for the claim that, for the common good of society (and of the human species), efficacy trials for HIV candidate vaccines should be undertaken as soon as possible. Some researchers argue that this is especially true given the fact that we do already have available candidate vaccines that have proven to be both safe and immunogenic (as we will see later). Some viral subunit candidate vaccines have even been proven partially efficacious in some animal models.

Given these considerations, say some researchers, it would seem grossly unethical to continue postponing these trials, especially in developing nations which are themselves anxious to have the trials take place among their own populations.

In other words, say Thesis proponents, we must consider the ethics of waiting. To wait, after all, is an act, an act that has consequences, and in this case it has severe consequences. If we choose to not support the Thesis position, and to instead recommend delay of the trials, then we should be aware that that choice will be attended by costs, and they are costs that deserve our serious attention.

These reasons lead us to the conclusion that we must not delay initiation of HIV vaccine trials any longer; rather, we must boldly go forward with them. The longer we wait, the greater the tragic cost will be.

If the Thesis position primarily urges boldness and moving ahead toward finding a safe and effective vaccine, out of a deep concern for the protection of those not yet infected, the Antithesis position primarily urges caution, reflection, wariness of haste; it urges a profound concern for the well-being of those tens of thousands of volunteers who will probably be participating in the trials.

The Antithesis position holds that we must, under no circumstances, begin phase I, II, or III HIV vaccine trials until we can insure that the individual rights and well-being of all volunteers will be protected to the fullest extent possible, as required by *The Nuremberg Code* and the WHO/CIOMS *Ethical Guidelines.*

In order to get a brief glimpse of some of the ethical issues raised by those who hold the Antithesis position, consider this one question (among numerous others that could equally well be posed):

> Why would any sensible, even moderately self-interested person ever consent to participate in experiments which entail the potential for so much risk to their personal health and their social well-being, and which have so little potential for any personal benefit? Might the reasons be that perhaps they simply have not been made fully aware of the degree of risk involved? Perhaps they were not fully informed by researchers? Or if they did participate in an "informing session," perhaps the information they were given did not register with them; perhaps they did not fully understand what they were told? Or perhaps they were, in some subtle way, deluded into thinking there would be some potential benefit to them in the form of possible

protection against HIV infection? Perhaps they were offered some inducement, by research sponsors, to participate? Perhaps they were in some way persuaded, or pressured, or possibly even coerced into participation by someone at the institution where the research is being conducted. Perhaps they were pressured or coerced by government or community leaders, or perhaps even by someone else close to them, such as a spouse or boss. When there is so much to potentially lose, and almost no likelihood of any personal benefit, why would anyone choose to volunteer for such trials?

These questions, and numerous others like them, are raised by those who hold the Antithesis position. They insist that it would probably be illegal, that it would certainly be immoral, and that it would likely have disastrous consequences for future research protocols if trials were to be initiated without fully adequate compliance with all requisite ethical guidelines.

In the largest sections of this book I will be primarily exploring and defending the point of view expressed by the Antithesis position, though it will be the task of this book to lay out the reasoning, the concepts, and the information that lie behind both of these positions. It is hoped that when the full force of the Thesis and Antithesis positions are more clearly understood, then the chances for a viable Synthesis position to emerge will become more promising.

Ethicists and researchers at the World Health Organization in Geneva and at the National Institutes of Health in the US have already been discussing these issues, of course, but as of the spring of 1996 many of the issues are still undecided and remain quite controversial. Educated citizens of the world community will want to be aware of the enormity of the decisions being faced. I intend this book to foster public discussion about these issues.

Most of the ethical quandaries discussed in this book will be understood only by the reader's having some prior familiarity with:

1 the present state of the HIV/AIDS pandemic, and its predicted future course;
2 some characteristics of the human immunodeficiency virus (HIV);
3 the basic nature of the human immune system; and
4 the various kinds of vaccines and how they work.

Accordingly, this book can be seen as having three main parts: the first chapters (1–7) outline some of these essential concepts and some of the basic (and more recent) information necessary for appreciating the ethical issues. Any adequate understanding of the two positions, particularly of the Thesis position, requires familiarity with the concepts and information in these chapters.

The central chapters in the book (8–23) then lay out some of the ethical difficulties faced by those who would wish to test HIV vaccines for use in human populations. This portion of the book is more representative of the Antithesis position, and details some of the operative ethical principles that ethicists use in assessing biomedical research. Some of the potential risks to research subjects are outlined, as well as some of the potential motivations which subjects might have for participating in these trials. This portion of the book also describes some of the problems involved in obtaining ethically appropriate informed consent from prospective subjects, problems with improper inducement of volunteers to participate in the trials, and issues relating to the problems of compensating volunteers for injuries suffered as a result of their participation in the studies.

A brief sampling of some of the questions raised in this section would include the following:

> How will researchers be able to execute an ethically adequate informed consent procedure when the amount of information necessary for subjects to understand is so great and the nature of it so complicated? How will researchers be able to provide information about the nature of vaccines and immune responses to persons (particularly in developing nations) who may hold conceptions of disease and disease-causality that are quite different from the conceptions of disease held by the researchers? How can research sponsors properly assess whether prospective subjects

have understood enough information so that they are able to give adequately informed consent? How can research counselors effectively counsel subjects to not engage in risky behaviors when they themselves realize, at some level, that the research protocol itself requires that subjects do engage in those risk behaviors? What are some of the potential harms that might reasonably be expected to accrue to subjects who participate in these trials, and what are some benefits they might theoretically expect which could counterbalance the risks they could be taking? What is to be done about protecting volunteers' confidentiality, and how can these volunteers be protected against unfair discrimination based on their new serostatus which will (often) result from their participation in the studies?

And underlying all these specific questions are deeper meta-questions, such as:

> Should the main operative ethical principles in this international vaccine research be different in different countries, varying according to the particular mores and cultural standards in each country, or should there be a set of common, agreed-upon international ethical standards for the protection of research subjects, applicable to all research protocols regardless of the country in which the research is conducted?

These questions and numerous others related to them, usually raised by persons sympathetic to the Antithesis position, will not be easy to deal with, nor will the answers to them be simple.

The final chapters of the book (24–27) offer one or two metaphors and some concluding suggestions for guiding our thinking about these difficult and yet unresolved complex questions. Another of my books (*Jenner on Trial: An Ethical Examination of Vaccine Research in the Age of Smallpox and The Age of AIDS*) also offers suggestions for how best to approach these difficult ethical questions concerning vaccine research.

People sometimes ask me which of the two key positions represented in this book, the Thesis position or the Antithesis position, I am personally more inclined toward holding. The simple answer to this question is that I see the validity in both positions, and that I am hoping a viable Synthesis position will emerge very soon.

The more complicated answer, however, would go something like this: I am a friend of the Thesis position. It seems to me that all the principles of human compassion require that we do everything in our power to find some truly effective ways to prevent any new infections with a microbe that causes such devastating personal disease and social havoc. Vaccines have traditionally been by far the most effective public health intervention ever devised – probably excepting only the provision of clean water – for preventing infectious disease. If there is any hope at all for developing an effective vaccine against this terrible disease, we should put enormous resources into doing so.

However, HIV vaccine trials will also pose ethical difficulties on a scale never before faced by biomedical researchers, and those ethical difficulties must be thoughtfully and thoroughly addressed as well.

In the Roman Catholic tradition, when the name of a (deceased) holy person is brought before the canonization tribunal to determine whether that person should be officially counted among the blessed, the process which the tribunal goes through for determining sainthood is both lengthy and thorough. The Church goes to such great lengths because she considers the matter of canonization to be of the highest importance. As all the evidence is being gathered to support the naming of this candidate to sainthood, one church official in the tribunal is assigned the contrary task of arguing that the candidate under consideration for sainthood should not be canonized. This official's job, while all the others on the tribunal are weighing evidence that favors canonization, is to find as much evidence and as many reasons as possible that count against this candidate's canonization.

The church's thinking is that the efforts of such an official – traditionally designated the "devil's advocate" – help insure that, if the candidate for sainthood is eventually canonized, the canonization process will have been performed as thoroughly and as critically as is humanly possible.

I see my own position as in some ways analogous to that of the devil's advocate: just as he favors a valid canonization, so I too favor the rapid development of a safe and effective vaccine to protect against what is probably the most devastating personal and communal disease of our era (so far). I see myself as a friend of the Thesis efforts, but as a friend who is temporarily voicing the arguments for the opposition; as a friend who wants to help insure that one position prevails, and is trying to help it prevail by opposing it.

I take this position for two reasons: first, because it seems clear to me that the arguments supporting the Thesis position are so strong, so cogent and so convincing to intelligent, informed persons of good will, that we need to insure that the arguments of the opposing position are heard as well. Secondly, those who presently hold the Thesis position will ultimately be required (primarily by Ethics Review Committees) to answer the arguments urged by those who hold the Antithesis position. Therefore it will be best if they can hear these arguments presented in as clear and persuasive a manner as possible.

The issues involved in the planning of international HIV vaccine efficacy trials are difficult and serious. "It is anticipated that such trials will be large and complex undertakings, and probable that several trials will be necessary."[7] Thousands, hundreds of thousands, and perhaps eventually millions, of human lives will be directly affected by the decisions we make in the next few years.

Readers are urged, therefore, to give these matters the full good judgment they deserve.

NOTES

1. D. F. Hoth, et al., "HIV Vaccine Development: *A Progress Report*", *Annals of Internal Medicine,* 8, 7.15 October (1994) 603–11., p 608.
2. J. Green. "Who Put the Lid on gp120?" *New York Times Magazine,* 26 March 1995: 50–57, 74, 82.
3. Reuters. "WHO Approves Large-Scale AIDS Vaccine Trials." *Centers for Disease Control AIDS Daily Update,* 14 October 1994. This story was actually mistaken in one particular: the three countries where the first large scale vaccine trials will probably occur are Brazil, Uganda, and Thailand, not Tanzania as the article said in the original.

The phase I and II trials have already begun in Bankok.

"Thirty recovering intravenous drug users today received the first dose of a vaccine being tested to see if it can guard against AIDS. . . . The purpose of the study is to see whether genetically engineered gp120 can produce necessary antibodies to guard against acquired immune deficiency syndrome. Questions have been raised in Thailand and abroad over the trials in part because the vaccine treats a strain of HIV that is not the one most commonly found among intravenous drug users in Thailand." Reuters. "WHO Approves Large-Scale AIDS Vaccine Trials." *Centers for Disease Control AIDS Daily Update,* 14 October 1994.

4. These two positions, while clearly opposed to each other, are not strictly mutually exclusive.
5. J. Mann and D. Tarantola. *AIDS in the World: Redefining the Global HIV/AIDS Pandemic* (New York: Oxford University Press, 1995, in press) 12.
6. M. Lappé. *Evolutionary Medicine: Rethinking the Origins of Disease* (San Francisco, CA: Sierra Club Books, 1994) 255+xii., p 109.
7. W. L. Heyward, et al., "Preparation for Phase III HIV vaccine efficacy trials: methods for the determination of HIV incidence", *AIDS,* 8, 9. September (1994) 1285–91., p 1285.

1 Where Stands the Pandemic Now?

The Thesis position urges that "In the face of so much growing personal tragedy associated with HIV infection, and in the face of such a rapidly expanding global pandemic, waiting any longer to initiate phase I and II trials for HIV vaccines would simply be wrong." In order to have any notion of the full force of this claim, we will need to have some elementary understanding of the present scope and predicted future course of the HIV/AIDS pandemic.

It is difficult, however, to convey any full sense of the enormity of a pandemic.

Because it is so difficult, I often ask students in my courses on Medical Ethics and the AIDS pandemic to read Daniel Defoe's *A Journal of the Plague Year.* In this novel the impact of the Black Death in London that year (1665) comes across most clearly in the day to day details. We see infected mothers and their children shut up inside their houses, with guards stationed in front to insure that they do not come out. We see carts full of bodies being wheeled off in the early morning hours to stinking mass graves just outside town. We see the weekly mortality sheets recording the numbers of dead for the previous week. We see people packing their goods into a cart and leaving town to live elsewhere if they can afford to do so. We see people losing faith in their God, and then we see others believing even more strongly and praying even more fervently than they prayed to their God before. We see individuals responding daily to the threat of coming down with a mortal sickness that they've seen their friends and family members die of only days ago. We see people who are healthy today coming down with the sickness and dying before tomorrow's supper. These daily details bring home to readers the impact of living in the midst of an epidemic of lethal infectious disease.

Similarly, daily details of what it is like to live in the midst of the AIDS pandemic can be seen in the daily events recorded in biographical and autobiographical writings of people like Robert O'Boyle,[1] Paul Monette,[2] Barbara Peabody,[3] Anne Richardson, Dietmar Bolle,[4] and countless others who have effectively chronicled their own and others' personal experiences with AIDS. It is these personal accounts of living with a new truth (or perhaps with an old truth never before fully understood) that bring the reality of the epidemic alive for us. These authors do an enormous service for those who do not live directly in the front lines of the pandemic.

Yet at some point the impact of the pandemic must be somehow reduced to numbers, laid out in the stark black suit of quantity, if we are ever to adequately characterize its scope.

The Tenth International Conference on AIDS, held in Yokohama in August of 1994, tried to do just that. During that conference, the following summary of the pandemic's extent and demography was distributed by Dr Jonathan Mann (Director of the Global AIDS Policy Coalition at Harvard, and first Director of the World Health Organization's Global Programme on AIDS) and Daniel Tarantola, also of Harvard's GAPC. The numbers are stark and the passage is lengthy, but please read these data carefully. The statistics tell a powerful story.

> As of 1 January 1994, the Global AIDS Policy Coalition estimated that 22.2 million people worldwide had been infected with HIV since the beginning of the pandemic. Of these, 20 million were adults (11.3 million men and 8.7 million women) and 2.2 million were children. The largest numbers of HIV-infected people were in sub-Saharan Africa (15.5 million; 70 percent of global total) and Southeast Asia (3 million; 14 percent). The number of HIV-infected people in Southeast Asia now exceeds the total of infected people in the entire industrialized world. Thus, the large majority of HIV infections (20.2 million; 91 percent) have occurred in the developing world. Worldwide, an estimated 16.2 million people were living with HIV or AIDS on 1 January 1994.
>
> The global total of cumulative HIV infections in adults has more than doubled in four years, from nearly 10 million in 1990 to 20 million in 1994. . . .

> During 1993, over 3.7 million new infections occurred worldwide in adults and children – over 10,000 a day. Sub-Saharan Africa contributed 1.8 million infections (49 percent) to the global total and Southeast Asia had 1.5 million (40 percent). During 1993, the industrialized world accounted for over 200,000 new infections (6 percent); clearly the burden of new HIV infections is increasingly borne by developing countries (over 3.5 million, or 94 percent). Globally, during 1993, 1.4 million women were newly infected, representing 40 percent of all new adult infections that year. . . .
>
> Globally, during 1993, over 350,000 children were born with HIV infection. . . .
>
> The epidemic has not been stopped in any country; the cumulative number of HIV infections continues to rise relentlessly. . . .
>
> The gap between the expanding pandemic and the response is growing rapidly and dangerously, [and] efforts in prevention and care are becoming fragmented. . . .
>
> [T]he current global AIDS strategy . . . is not sufficient to meet the challenges of the pandemic. . . .[5]

In Thailand, for example, as in some other developing countries, the epidemic is almost out of control. The infection rate, says Dr Prayura Kunasol, head of Thailand's Department of Communicable Disease Control, "has hit 20 percent among young military recruits – and 8 per cent amount pregnant women – in the country's northern Chang Mai province. AIDS patients now occupy half of Chang Mai's hospital beds".[6]

Although HIV began to spread widely in Thailand only as recently as 1987, already infection levels are approaching 23 per cent of the reproductive age population.[7] The three factors that are largely responsible for this discouraging situation in Thailand are: a) the rapid growth of HIV infection nationwide, b) the fact that infection is not limited to identifiable "risk groups" (e.g., gay men or injection drug users) but is spread throughout the "general population," and c) the presence of a large infected but still symptom-free (hence unidentifiable) population of HIV carriers, most of whom do not realize that they are infected, and who will then probably be spreading the virus to their sex partners. HIV positive women who become pregnant also risk spreading the infection to their fetuses. These three features are not unique to Thailand, but actually characterize many Asian countries.[8]

In India, for example, "studies have documented infection rates of 50–75 percent among IV-drug users in some provinces", and in Bombay "the rate [of HIV infection] among prospective blood donors shot from less than 1 percent in 1992 to 5 percent last year". This figure has tremendous consequences for protecting the quality of the national blood supply, especially since in India blood-testing facilities outside of major cities are rare.[9] India simply cannot afford to test any more than a small fraction of blood donations at present.[10]

Nor are India and Thailand unique. Drug use, commercial sex and general ignorance about the risks of HIV transmission unfortunately are commonplace in many countries, both industrial and developing.[11] Economic difficulties exacerbate the problems. Cambodia, for example, does indeed have a national AIDS prevention program, but it has not been implemented because of lack of funding.[12]

These examples are from Asia, but the situation in South America is not much better, and the situation in Africa is very much worse. No statistic tells it as clearly as this one: "Less than ten per cent of the world's population but more than 60 per cent of the world's HIV-infected people are African."[13]

Thus, if we had to sum up the state of the global epidemic so far, we would have to say that it is getting worse by the day. In the US it is estimated that there is one new HIV infection every 9 or 10 minutes.[14] That statistic, tragic though it is, is not as dramatic as the statistics for the whole globe. When I began teaching courses on Medical Ethics and AIDS in 1987, I could accurately tell students that, according to the most current data, there was a new HIV infection somewhere in the world every 30 seconds. A few years later I could tell students that there was one new infection every 20 seconds. When I taught the course in early 1994 I could tell them there was a new infection every 10 seconds. According to the figures above which were released at the Yokohama conference, there is now a new HIV infection somewhere in the world every 8.5 seconds.

Nor do these numbers take into account the dramatic resurgence of "the white plague," tuberculosis, which has been recrudescing in direct proportion to the global increase in HIV disease. HIV disease, or in fact any immunodeficiency condition regardless of its cause, is a direct correlate to the increase in active TB cases. In fact, of all the opportunistic infections associated with AIDS, tuberculosis is the most common, worldwide, and is the only OI that puts non-HIV-infected persons at any significant risk.

What is also true, though not so commonly known, is that the presence of active tuberculosis infection (indeed, the presence of any active mycobacterium infection) in an individual HIV+ person appears to speed the progress of HIV infection in that individual so that they proceed to active AIDS much more rapidly. It can be said, therefore, that HIV is a catalyst for the increase of TB in a community, and that TB is a catalyst for the increase of AIDS both in individuals and in communities.[15]

This is indeed a bleak picture of an epidemic that C. Everett Koop, former US Surgeon General, has called "the number one health problem on this planet".[16]

Epidemiological statistics are not, of course, the only measure of an epidemic. AIDS, we have discovered, is at least as much a social, political, and economic problem as it is a medical problem. In fact every major epidemic is a social and political problem as much as it is a medical problem. Writing in 1976, five years before the first case of AIDS had been noticed or identified, historian William McNeill tried to describe the effects of epidemics in past ages:

> The disruptive effect of . . . epidemic[s] is likely to be greater than the mere loss of life, severe as that may be. Often survivors are demoralized, and lose all faith in inherited custom and belief which had not prepared them for such a disaster. . . . Population losses within the twenty to forty age bracket are obviously far more damaging to society at large than comparably numerous destruction of either the

very young or the very old. Indeed, any community that loses a substantial percentage of its young adults in a single epidemic finds it hard to maintain itself materially and spiritually. When an initial exposure to one civilized infection is swiftly followed by similarly destructive exposure to others, the structural cohesion of the community is almost certain to collapse.[17]

His concern is shared by others. Susan Sontag, in her literary study, *AIDS and Its Metaphors*, quotes a German AIDS specialist, Dr Eike Brigitte Helm, who says that "in a number of parts of the world AIDS will drastically change the population structure. Particularly in Africa and Latin America. A society that is not able, somehow or other, to prevent the spread of AIDS has very poor prospects for the future."[18] Then Jonathan Mann tells us that in fact not one society so far has succeeded in preventing the spread of AIDS. "No community or country in the world already affected by AIDS can claim that HIV spread has stopped."[19]

We have here, it seems, the makings of a syllogism. It looks something like this:

Premise: Any society that cannot prevent the spread of AIDS has very poor prospects for the future.

Premise: Every society already affected by AIDS has failed to prevent the spread of AIDS.

The conclusion to this little syllogism would seem to be momentous:

Every society already affected by AIDS has poor prospects for the future.

A conclusion of this sort may perhaps be hyperbolic for some societies, but is probably an accurate conclusion for others.

In underdeveloped communities, for example, whether in developing nations or developed nations, AIDS is expected to have widespread devastating consequences. Social structures and economic support systems in these communities have less "give" in them because there are fewer redundant systems to use for backup when a main system fails. Furthermore, because AIDS strikes at the young adult population, i.e., at those persons in a society who are producing a large per cent of the goods and services for the community, and who are also the parents and breadwinners in families, the economic consequences to these societies, which are already severe, are only expected to get worse.

There may be labor shortages, for example, and these shortages could slow down or even reverse recent development gains. Furthermore, "economies may be further damaged by declines in foreign investment or by a drying up of tourism. In many Asian societies, the elderly are dependent on their working sons and daughters for support. When their children die, not only will the elderly often find themselves unsupported, but they may have to take responsibility for their orphaned grandchildren."[20] Thus, the direct impact on families and on the raising of children (who are the community's future) can be expected to be significant.

Globally, in economic terms, the costs are surprisingly large. The United Nations *Human Development Report 1994* features a prominent sidebar titled "HIV and AIDS – a global epidemic," in which is summarized some of the information you've just read. Then they present some calculations of economic impact. Costs of the epidemic, of course, include a wide variety of factors. There are direct medical and hospitalization costs, research costs, prevention costs, public health program costs, education costs, and many others, and there are also the indirect costs of years of potential life lost (YPLL), of lost productivity, and of the further consequent economic fallout from that lost productivity. The United Nations Development Programme attempted to quantify these costs. They calculated some conservative estimates of what these costs have totaled to date, and what they might be expected to rise to in the future. Here are their figures:

> The cumulative direct and indirect costs of HIV and AIDS in the 1980s have been conservatively estimated at $240 billion. The social and psychological costs of the epidemic for individuals, families, communities and nations are also huge – but inestimable. . . .
>
> The global cost – direct and indirect – of HIV and AIDS by 2000 could be as high as $500 billion *a year* – equivalent to more than 2% of global GDP.[21]

This conservative estimate of the annual costs of this pandemic by the year 2000, only three years away, is staggering and can be expected to have serious economic implications for the whole globe. It certainly lends credence to the assertion that something must be done to stem the problem. The epidemic does not look like it will go away on its own.

The United Nations has once again recognized the world wide impact of this pandemic and has announced a major reorganization of its global efforts at controlling the disease. In place of WHO's Global Programme on AIDS (which no longer exists), there now is an overall, high-level coordinating agency called the Joint United Nations Programme on HIV/AIDS (UNAIDS), headed by Belgian scientist, Dr Peter Piot, that has the function of bringing together and focusing the efforts of all the various United Nations agencies that deal with AIDS.[22] UN agencies that currently deal with AIDS include the World Health Organization, the United Nations Development Program (UNDP), the United Nations Population Fund (UNFPA), UNESCO, UNICEF, and the World Bank. (The UN is to be applauded for its long recognition that AIDS, in addition to its dimension as a medical problem, is also a social, economic, educational, research and political problem as well.) The announcement of this major organizational change in WHO's approach to the AIDS pandemic marked

> the first time in the 50-year history of the UN that any disease or health crisis has been elevated to such a level. This is occurring because the international community has never before faced such an intractable, rapidly expanding and economically costly new disease crisis.[23]

To sum up, the social, psychological, public health, and economic consequences from this epidemic are already tragic, and are expected to become much more severe in many parts of the world. The Thesis position holds that something dramatic must be done soon.

NOTES

1. R. O'Boyle. *Living With AIDS* (Seattle, WA: *The Seattle Times*, 1992) 62.
2. P. Monette. *Borrowed Time* (New York, NY: Avon, 1988) 342.
3. B. Peabody. *The Screaming Room* (New York, NY: Avon, 1986) 279.
4. A. Richardson and D. Bolle, eds. *Wise Before Their Time: People from Around the World Living with AIDS and HIV Tell Their Stories* (London: Harper Collins, 1992) 144.
5. Mann, Jonathan, and Daniel Tarantola, eds. *AIDS in the World: Redefining the Global HIV/AIDS Pandemic* (New York: Oxford University Press) forthcoming, 12. pp 1–3.
6. G. Cowley and M. Hager. "The Ever-Expanding Plague." *Newsweek* 22 August 1994: 37.
7. T. Brown and P. Xenos. "AIDS: Epidemic in Asia." *Seattle Post-Intelligencer* 2 October 1994. D1, D3.
8. *Ibid.*
9. Cowley, Geoffrey, and Mary Hager. "The Ever-Expanding Plague." *Newsweek* 22 August 1994: 37.
10. T. Brown and P. Xenos. "AIDS: Epidemic in Asia." *Seattle Post-Intelligencer* 2 October 1994. D1, D3.

    India is not unique in its inadequately screened blood supply. Some parts of Africa have serious problems also: "even after blood screening, the risk of a unit of blood in Abidjan being HIV-infected was estimated to be at least 5.4 per 1000 units, grater than the risk in Europe or North America before the introduction of HIV testing." K. M. De Cock MD, MRCP, DTM&H, et al., "The Public Health Implications of AIDS Research in Africa", *JAMA*, 272, 6.10 August (1994) 481–86., p 483.
11. Just for the sake of clarification, the United Nations Development Program (UNDP) formally defines nations as falling within one of three categories: high development, medium development, and low development. Low development nations are those whose Human Development Index (HDI) has a value of .500 or below. Medium development countries are those whose HDI has a value of .501 to .799. Highly developed countries are those whose HDI is .800 to 1.00. For a full discussion of the wide range of factors that are considered in the HDI see M. ul Haq, ed. *Human Development Report 1994* (New York, NY: Oxford University Press, 1994) 226+xii.
12. T. Brown and P. Xenos. "AIDS: Epidemic in Asia." *Seattle Post-Intelligencer* 2 October 1994. D1, D3.
13. K. M. De Cock MD, MRCP, DTM&H, et al., "The Public Health Implications of AIDS Research in Africa", *JAMA*, 272, 6.10 August (1994) 481–86., p 485.
14. D. F. Hoth, et al., "HIV Vaccine Development: A Progress Report", *Annals of Internal Medicine*, 8, 7.15 October (1994) 603–11., p 603.
15 The global increase in tuberculosis, while directly related to the increase of HIV infection and AIDS, and while it dramatically exacerbates the health problems in any community that is affected by AIDS, is not directly related to the central issues raised in this book.

I mention tuberculosis here only to underline the multidimensionality and the severity of the HIV/AIDS pandemic. See F. Ryan MD. *The Forgotten Plague: How the Battle Against Tuberculosis was Won – and Lost* (published in England as *The Greatest Story Never Told*) of (Boston: Little, Brown and Co, 1992, 1993) 460+xx.

A significant difficulty that results from the increasing prevalence of both tuberculosis and HIV infection, and the fact that each seems to potentiate the other, is that public health officials must now re-evaluate whether to continue administering BCG vaccine for tuberculosis, since the live, attenuated virus that makes up the TB vaccine may also interact with HIV in those who are HIV+. This is only one example of how HIV complicates the public health picture in the world in ways that we may not fully understand for quite some time. See J. R. Starke and K. K. Connelly. "Bacille Calmette-Guérin Vaccine." *Vaccines.* Eds. Stanley A. Plotkin MD and Edward A. Mortimer Jr, MD, second ed. (Philadelphia: W.B. Saunders Company, 1994) 439–73., p 464.

16. UPI. In *Seattle Post-Intelligencer,* 28 January 1988.
17. W. H. McNeill. *Plagues and Peoples* (Garden City, NY: Doubleday Anchor, 1976) 340+xii., p 61.
18. S. Sontag. *AIDS and Its Metaphors* (New York: Farrar, Straus and Giroux, 1988) 95, p 91.

Consider also:

> [T]his pandemic will have profound economic and social implications for both developed and developing countries. The importance of health as an input to the economic development and growth of a country is well established – a healthier population is more productive and has an increased capacity for learning. The adverse impacts of the HIV/AIDS pandemic will undermine improvements in health status and, in turn, reduce the potential for economic growth. AIDS is distinct from other diseases, and its impact can be expected to be quite severe. . . . Its most critical feature, distinguishing AIDS from other life-threatening and fatal illnesses, such as diarrhea (among children in developing countries) or cancer (among the elderly in developed countries), is that it selectively affects adults in their sexually most active ages, which coincide with their prime productive and reproductive years. Jill Armstrong, an economist in the Eastern Africa Dept of the World Bank, and Eduard Bos, a demographer in the Population, Health, and Nutrition Division of the World Bank's Population and Human Resources Department. Quoted in Mann, Jonathan (General Editor), Daniel Tarantola (Scientific Editor), and Thomas Netter (Managing Editor), *AIDS in the World* (Cambridge, MA: Harvard University Press, 1992) 1037+xvi, p 195.

See also Appendix IV on the effects of AIDS in developing nations.

19. J. Mann, D. Tarantola and T. Netter, eds. *AIDS in the World* (Cambridge, MA: Harvard University Press, 1992) 1037+xvi., p 2.

20. T. Brown and P. Xenos. "AIDS: Epidemic in Asia." *Seattle Post-Intelligencer* 2 October 1994. D1, D3.
21. UNDP. *Human Development Report 1994* (United Nations Development Programme, 1994) UNDP, p 28. Emphasis mine.
22. M. Balter, "UN Readies New Global AIDS Plan", *Science,* 266.25 November (1994) 1312–13., p 1312.
23. L. Garrett. "Unified AIDS Fight; UN combines agency efforts." *Newsday* 13 December 1994. A37.

    Coincidentally, the US Centers for Disease Control and Prevention has also announced a major restructuring of its AIDS-control efforts. See L. Thompson, "CDC Reorganization Prompts Concern", *Science,* 266.25 November (1994) 1313.

2 It's Not Just Another Disease

Furthermore, urges the Thesis position, the uniqueness of this disease makes it an especially formidable enemy, and one that will be particularly difficult to get under any semblance of control.

This is the case because the more we learn about this disease, the more we are learning that "whatever else AIDS is, it is not just another disease," says Dr June Osborn, past chair of the US National Commission on AIDS. Nor is AIDS just another epidemic, nor even just another global pandemic. Several features of this disease make it unique among diseases, and unique among epidemics.

2.1 HIGH MORBIDITY AND MORTALITY

We are dealing with a disease that has an exceptionally high degree of morbidity and mortality. It has been conservatively estimated that 90 per cent, perhaps more, of those who become infected with HIV will eventually contract AIDS and die of it.[1] This conservative estimate is considered quite significant; very few microbes kill as many as 50 per cent of those they infect.[2]

2.2 LIFELONG INFECTIOUSNESS

We are dealing with a disease that is life long. This means that HIV positive persons will be infectious for the rest of their lives. Not only is this an enormous burden of personal tragedy for them as individuals, but it also means that any behavioral changes required of them will need to be put into effect for the rest of their lives.

2.3 LENGTHY ASYMPTOMATIC STAGE

We are dealing with a disease that has an extremely long asymptomatic period – some call it a "latency" period – during which time the infected person shows no visible signs of infection, but is fully capable of passing the virus to anyone with whom blood or body fluids are shared. Of even more concern to some is the fact that during the first several weeks immediately following the new infection, none of the commonly used tests for detecting HIV infection will be able to detect that there has been a new infection. Therefore, newly infected persons do not have any way of detecting whether or not they have become infected with HIV, and consequently, neither do their sexual partners have any way of knowing whether their partner has been infected. And now recent evidence suggests that during those first 4–6 weeks immediately following a new infection, the newly infected person is especially contagious to others. In other words, "people are extremely contagious in the first 60 days after getting [HIV] – the same period in which they don't [yet] know they have it".[3]

Furthermore, except for getting tested, there are no obvious signs of infection visible for years, perhaps up to ten or more years. There is no visible evidence at all that a person might be infected with HIV. This means that infected persons themselves may have no idea that they are infected, and certainly no one looking at them would have any reason to think they are infected.

One of the many consequences of this reality is that the success of any prevention measures we take now will not be evident for many years to come. This poses a serious public health problem because when there is such a long period of time between cause and effect (between HIV infection and AIDS), it is difficult for people to see any real connection between their behavior now and the possible consequences many years later. This makes it difficult to motivate people (or governments) to take preventive precautions.

2.4 HIGHLY MUTABLE

We are dealing with a virus which is highly mutable, which replicates rapidly and mutates often. This means that researchers and clinicians are aiming at a constantly moving target, a target that changes its coat almost every time it reproduces. (More on this in chapter 5 below.)

2.5 EFFECTIVE MODES OF TRANSMISSION

We are dealing with a virus that, by chance, has figured out some very effective ways of getting itself transmitted from one host to another. It is true that HIV is not transmitted by casual contact, (which is very good news) but some of the ways that it is transmitted – sexual contact, blood transfusion, birth, etc. – are fairly common behaviors. Many people have sexual contact with others, have blood transfusions, and all of us have been born. These are not unusual or abnormal behaviors. Of those who have so far been infected with HIV in the world, over 85 per cent have been infected via sexual contact.[4] When we add injection drug use to our list of modes of transmission, we see that between drug use and sexual activity, HIV gets itself transmitted from host to host by means of some of the most "biologically urgent" of human behaviors. They are also behaviors that are largely private, often pleasurable, and occasionally unlawful, which means that they are behaviors that are liable to be rather difficult to exert any social controls over. If a parasite (such as HIV) has to find some effective way to get from one host to another in order to insure its continued propagation, HIV has certainly found some very effective ways to do that.

2.6 DESTROYS THE IMMUNE SYSTEM

We are dealing with a disease which, unlike almost any other, targets the immune system itself, and destroys the very system whose purpose it is to protect us from disease. Furthermore, HIV targets and kills one of the key cells in the immune system, the T4 cell (or CD4 cell), which orders and orchestrates the whole cellular and humoral immune response. When these T4 cells are destroyed, the immune system itself is destroyed.

2.7 VIRAL RESERVOIR EXPANDING

As the epidemic continues to grow in numbers and extent, i.e., as the total number of infected persons grows daily, the total quantity of HIV on the planet is also growing daily. This means that "the reservoir of infection, i.e., the total sum of people infected who can also act as a source of infectious virus to others, is also constantly and progressively expanding".[5] This has the total overall effect of amplifying the spread of infection. The faster it spreads, the faster it spreads.

These seven features of the disease make it a particularly formidable opponent. Dr Barry D Schoub, Director of the National Institute of Virology at the University of Witwatersrand in Johannesburg, sums up the matter thus:

> [T]he ability of the virus to cause a slow, progressive and permanent infection with permanent infectivity makes it a unique cause of epidemic disease. Thus, with no recovery, no loss of infectivity, no development of either individual or herd immunity, there is no known biological mechanism which can stop the continuing expansion of the disease unless an effective vaccine were to come about, and at present there is no feasible design for such an effective vaccine. The progressive increase in the pool of HIV can, in theory, only lead to an exponential increase in the number of individuals who will become infected until eventually the majority of the sexually active population will be infected unless interventions are at lease moderately successful.[6]

Given a disease with these particular characteristics, it is small wonder that this epidemic is growing at the rate it is. All reliable evidence indicates that, for as far into the future as we can presently reliably estimate, the pandemic will probably continue to grow at its present, or even perhaps at an accelerating, rate.

NOTES

1. R. Berkow and A. J. Fletcher, eds. *The Merck Manual of Diagnosis and Therapy*. Fifteenth ed. (Rahway, NJ: Merck Sharp & Dohme Research Laboratories, 1987) 2697+xxviii., p 292.
2. L. Garrett. *The Coming Plague: Newly Emerging Diseases in a World Out of Balance* (New York, NY: Farrar, Straus and Giroux, 1994) 750+xiv., p 20.
3. "The data suggest that rates of HIV infection during that early period may be 100 to 1,000 times higher than in the long asymptomatic phase that follows." K. Fackelmann, "HIV's infectious nature", *Science News*, 14 January (1995) 22.

   Also Knight-Ridder-Newspapers. "AIDS extremely contagious in early stages, study finds." *The Seattle Times* 6 January 1995. A7.
4. J. Mann, D. Tarantola and T. Netter, eds. *AIDS in the World* (Cambridge, MA: Harvard University Press, 1992) 1037+xvi. p 33.
5. B. D. Schoub. *AIDS & HIV in Perspective* (New York, NY: Cambridge University Press, 1994) 268+xx., p 17.
6. *Ibid.* p 244.

3 Will it Ever Slow Down?

An accelerating epidemic of this proportion (of "biblical proportions," says one AIDS expert[1]) does not just go away. Four possible developments, however, could make this epidemic diminish:

1 We could find a cure.
2 Human behaviors could radically change.
3 The virus could become weaker.
4 We could develop a preventive vaccine.

Each of these possibilities deserves a lengthy discussion, but this book will briefly skim over three of them and focus attention on the fourth, the preventive vaccine.

3.1 A CURE?

A cure is not to hold your breath for. In the past 50 years it is true that scientific medicine has developed cures for a wide range of infectious agents, but none of these have been viral agents. We have no cures for any diseases caused by viruses. Our ability to get some viral diseases under control, even eliminated, has been due more to preventive vaccines than to any other factor. Nobel laureate Joshua Lederberg explains why it is that we are able to cure bacterial diseases – i.e., why we are able to kill bacteria – but are unable to cure viral diseases:

> [B]acteria are free-living organisms whose metabolic peculiarities lend themselves to differential attack. E.g., the bacterial cell wall is utterly unlike any structure found in human cells. Hence penicillin [or any other antibiotic] which attacks the integrity of the bacterial cell wall, is all but innocuous to human tissue, and can be given in very large doses so as to saturate every susceptible bacterial cell. Viruses, however, are genetic fragments which live within the host cells and exploit their metabolism. It has so far been very difficult to find chemicals that will inhibit

> a virus without harming the host cell at the same time. Our principal strategy for dealing with viruses is immunization, evoking antibodies that recognize the peculiarities of the virus surface. When a virus, like [HIV], comes along and targets the immune system itself, we are left with dimmer hopes of being able to use that strategy; and we have very few alternatives.[3]

None of the sources familiar to the author has reported a single knowledgeable expert who expects a cure in the foreseeable future. In fact at the Tenth International AIDS Conference in Yokohama, Dr Jay Levy, one of the world's leading researchers into the epidemic stated that "a cure for AIDS is virtually impossible by the end of this century".[4] One problem is HIV's ability to mutate into forms resistant to drugs, such as AZT, ddI, ddC and others, that have been used against it.[5] Even if it looked like a cure might be possible, its actual application would be so far in the future that the epidemic would have grown even more out of control than it is now (especially given the necessity for lengthy human clinical trials to establish safety and efficacy; such trials can take, even with the FDA's accelerated drug development procedure, ten years or more).

And while it is true that cure is more interesting than prevention (cures certainly win more headlines), there is much wisdom in the old cliché which claims that an ounce of prevention is worth a pound of cure.

In any case, it really does not look like a cure is going to be the way that this epidemic will be slowed down.

3.2 BEHAVIOR CHANGE?

What kinds of behavior changes would need to happen in order to get this epidemic slowed down or stopped? Some of the necessary behavior changes would include personal or individual changes, some would include broad cultural and societal changes, and some necessary changes would even include major transformations at the governmental, political, and even international levels.

3.2.1 Sex, drugs and human rights

Human behaviors, in the realm of sexual practices, both homosexual and heterosexual (over 70 per cent of HIV infections in the world are due to heterosexual transmission),[6] and in the realm of drug abuse (both recreational drugs and therapeutic drugs[7]), would have to radically change. The average number of sexual partners in a lifetime, for example, would have to be dramatically reduced, particularly in certain cultures and sub-cultures. The practice of actual, faithful monogamy (both homosexual and heterosexual) would need to become far more popular world-wide than it is now, especially in cultures and subcultures which presently encourage or treat as acceptable the idea of multiple sexual partners. The use of condoms and other prophylactic safer sex methods would need to increase dramatically. Injection drug use world-wide would need to markedly decrease, and the practice of injection drug users (IDUs) sharing drug injection equipment would need to cease. The number of drug treatment centers around the world would need to greatly increase so that "treatment on demand" could become a reality.

Necessary societal changes would also include a significant global shift in the social status of women, and in the ability of women to determine the particular circumstances of their lives. Women in many nations, for example, still have little say concerning economics, education, marriage, and other matters directly relating to their sexual lives, and hence have little or no power over their vulnerability to HIV infection.[8] As Jonathan Mann made clear at the Yokohama conference, issues of human rights must be given the highest priority if we are ever to get this pandemic under control.[9]

In addition, personal, cultural and national behaviors that lead to widespread global malnutrition would also need to radically change. There would have to be major improvements in blood supply screening, changes in a broad range of sanitation practices, and changes in a variety of other public health measures (including education) designed to increase the overall level of public health. And, unrelated as it may seem, the political instabilities of war, the political oppression of peoples, and the failure to protect and enforce economic rights are also enormously significant factors in the quality of international public health. Methods of resolving conflicts between enemy states must also undergo radical global change.[10]

All of this is a big order, of course, and deserves a great deal more discussion, though not in this book. Such a discussion, though, if we did explore it, would need to include the fact that, from a purely medical perspective, AIDS is a preventable disease. Researchers very early discovered that the most common modes of transmission – sexual practices and the sharing of drug injection equipment – all involve deliberate behaviors that in most cases could be consciously chosen, modified, or avoided. In this sense, HIV infection is largely preventable, at least at the level of the individual person. In this respect, HIV infection is unlike many other viral diseases that we vaccinate against, which are transmitted by casual contact and/or through the air.

In the case of HIV infection, however, one individual changing his or her sexual or drug-using behavior is an entirely different proposition than whole populations and whole cultures changing their commonly accepted behaviors. This fact, together with the political, social and public health factors listed above, make large scale social change of the sort that would be necessary, look less likely.

A cautious predictor of human behavior would perhaps say that change of this magnitude is a very tall order, and not likely to occur in the near future. Education alone certainly is not very likely to effect large scale behavioral change. Schoub says that

> On the wider global scale, education has been largely unsuccessful in effecting meaningful behaviour change, especially in the developing world. Of particular concern are the observations that, although education has often achieved a greater awareness in African populations, it has failed to translate this into appropriate modifications in behaviour. For example, a recent study in rural Uganda found that even though 86% of the surveyed population understood the nature of sexual transmission of HIV, nevertheless the HIV infection rate remained high. . . .[11]

Furthermore, improvement in the empowerment and social status of the world's women, particularly in some developing nations, is liable to be "a particularly difficult problem in the male-dominated societies of the developing world where poverty and ignorance have entrenched age-old cultural prejudices".[12]

Therefore, if large scale behavioral change is not very likely to happen in the near future, we will probably need to look elsewhere for ways to control the epidemic.

3.2.2 Quarantine?

One other possible public health measure for controlling epidemics should probably at least be mentioned in this context, if only to dismiss it, because it is sometimes brought up in discussions even among knowledgeable and reflective people. The measure I am referring to is the suggestion to isolate all HIV infected persons in their homes or in communes or compounds. That way, the argument goes, they would be much less likely to infect people outside the compound. "We used quarantine as a public health measure to control leprosy by containing lepers in leper colonies," says this proposal, "and we used isolation in TB sanatoria to control the spread of tuberculosis. Why can't we do the same with HIV+ people to control the spread of AIDS? If all HIV+ persons were off in their own communities, then the rest of us would not have to worry so much about becoming infected. After all, that's what they did in Cuba, isn't it? If it works there, why couldn't it work here?"

Just to briefly clarify the terminology, such a public health policy is actually more properly termed "isolation" than "quarantine". Quarantine is the practice that cities used to use during the years of the Black Death. When a ship from another country came into port, the city would require the ship and all its crew to stay on board out in the harbor for forty days (quarantine) before they allowed anyone from the ship to come ashore. That way the city would know that people on the ship, if they had not become sick during that forty days, were probably free of the plague and therefore would not bring disease to the city. Even during the outbreak of plague that occurred in India in the Fall of 1994, some international airports instituted a policy of quarantine for flights arriving into their airport from India. Ground crews were instructed to radio ahead to incoming pilots just as their plane was approaching the airport to ask if anyone on board had any evidence of bronchial infection (coughing, etc.). If the pilot answered yes, then the whole planeload of passengers was to be kept in a separate room in the airport for a period of two or three days to see if they developed plague, or if they instead just had ordinary colds or bronchial infections. This policy of quarantine was intended to prevent persons from India from bringing the plague into other countries.

Isolation, on the other hand, is the practice of separating infected persons off in their homes or in separate compounds so that they do not spread the infection to others in the wider community. Isolation has indeed been used as a public health practice for preventing the spread of infectious diseases in the past, but it would not be a useful method for controlling the spread of HIV infection for several reasons. And while it is true that Cuba did initiate such a policy and kept it in place for several years, that policy was abandoned in late 1993 as an overly expensive and ultimately ineffective method of infection control. Bulgaria too made a short attempt at isolation of HIV+ persons, but soon abandoned it as prohibitively expensive.[13] The reasons against the use of such a policy are basically three: a) it is extremely costly, b) it is ineffective, and c) it is an enormous and unnecessary abridgment of individual civil rights. Let's look at each reason briefly.

a It would be an extremely costly policy. In addition to the costs of establishing and maintaining entire separate communes or villages for HIV+ persons, there would be all the costs associated with regularly testing entire populations. HIV+ persons cannot be distinguished from HIV– persons except by testing, so the entire population of a country would need to be tested to discover which persons were HIV+. That would be such a horrendously expensive proposition that no one has seriously suggested that it be done. Furthermore, the number of false positives in such a broad population screening program would be extremely high, leading to accidental isolation of many HIV– persons too. Such HIV screening, furthermore, would need to be done every few months, perhaps even more often than that, which means the high costs would be continuous and ongoing. When we add to that the mammoth costs of the bureaucracy that would be needed to carry out such a program and to adjudicate all the disputes that would undoubtedly arise in connection with testing, we can see that policymakers would simply have to decide whether this was really how they wanted such a large percentage of their public health dollars to be spent.

b In addition to the false positives, there is also the problem of false negatives – i.e., people who are actually HIV antibody positive (HIVAb+) but test out as HIV antibody negative (HIVAb–). These are people who actually are infected with HIV, but whom the test says are not infected. This problem would mean that there are some HIV+ persons still in the community. Even more importantly, there is the matter of the lengthy "window period" – the time between actual HIV infection and the time when that infected person will test positive for the presence of antibodies. This window period can be several weeks long, sometimes as long as six months, and in rare cases as long as a year. People in this window period will test negative for the presence of HIVAb, but will still be actually infected with the virus and, of course, will be fully capable of infecting others. All these HIV+ persons would be missed in such a testing program and therefore could go on continuing to pass the virus to those with whom they have sexual or body fluid contact.

Also missed in such a mass screening program would be all those who simply slip through the cracks of the bureaucracy and do not get tested, for example persons who live largely outside the law, or who have no home address, who live on the streets, etc. There would also be a sizable number of persons who would try every trick and con they could think of (or afford) to avoid being tested. Many people would be very highly motivated to avoid such testing, so the abuses of the testing system would become significant, and would lead to even more costly attempts to enforce the policy and to resolve all the disputes that would arise as a result of the policy.

In other words, in addition to being an extremely costly public health measure, it would also be ineffective. Worse than that, it would seriously undermine (for no defensible reason) some of the basic liberties that many citizens feel are essential to the well-being of a liberal democratic state.

c Isolation would be an unnecessary abridgment of individual civil rights. Nations such as Cuba and Bulgaria, which do not have a strong tradition of protecting individual civil liberties, would find it easier to persuade the populace that such a practice is acceptable, and would find it easier to actually enforce such a policy. In a liberal democratic polity such as those found in Western Europe, the UK, North America, and elsewhere, however, policymakers would probably encounter a very high degree of resistance to the idea of isolating HIV+ individuals. Isolation would need to entail lengthy due process procedures to ensure that there are no abuses of the system. Citizens might feel that they would be living in something akin to a police state, so the potential for serious political rebellion would need to be considered as well.

All in all, I hear no one seriously proposing isolation of HIV+ persons as a way of controlling the AIDS pandemic. It would not work. It would be extraordinarily costly. It would abrogate more individual liberties than most people would be willing to tolerate, and all for no useful purpose. Even Cuba and Bulgaria, the only nations that even tried to experiment with such isolation, have given it up as useless.

Quarantine/isolation will hardly be the way that this pandemic is brought under control.

3.3 A WEAKER VIRUS?

Some optimistic thinkers hope that the human immunodeficiency virus might simply just moderate over time, perhaps becoming less infectious, or at least not causing the same severity of illness that it does now. If this were to happen, it would indeed be very good news. There do appear to have been some cases in the history of human-microbe interactions in which the microbe did mutate in such a way that it became less pathogenic to its human host.

Recent research suggests, however, that this is not a very likely outcome for HIV. In fact, it could be the case that in many, if not most, virus-host relationships, the tendency is for the microbe to mutate toward greater virulence.

> The general theme that virus-host relationships evolve toward less virulent, stable commensalism has been criticized by R M May & R M Anderson. . . . They stress that selection within the infected host favors the more virulent genotypes, however this may result in a deprivation of prey and further spread of the parasite.[14]

If HIV were indeed to mutate toward "greater virulence," what form might that greater virulence take? Several possibilities come to mind. Greater virulence could mean that persons who were infected with HIV would move more rapidly toward disease than they do now, within months, for example, rather than years. Or it could mean that the disease processes caused by HIV would be even more dreadful than they are now (though that might be difficult to imagine). Or it could mean that the mortality rate of HIV infection would increase to some rate even higher than it is now. Or it could mean that the sexual or blood-borne transmission of HIV from one host to another could become even more efficient than it is now. Or it could mean that HIV would develop the ability to be transmitted by new means that do not transmit it now. Joshua Lederberg considers, for example, the possibility of HIV "learning the tricks of airborne transmission:"

> We know that HIV is still evolving. Its global spread has meant there is far more HIV on earth today than ever before in history. What are the odds of its learning the tricks of airborne transmission? The short answer is "No one can be sure." . . . [A]s time passes, and HIV seems settled in a certain groove, that is momentary reassurance in itself. However, given its other ugly attributes, it is hard to imagine a worse threat to humanity than an airborne variant of AIDS. No rule of nature contradicts such a possibility; the proliferation of AIDS cases with secondary pneumonia [and TB] multiplies the odds of such a mutant, as an analog to the emergence of pneumonic plague.[15]

Whether HIV will mutate toward greater virulence or toward lesser virulence is still an open question, but it is clearly a question that deserves much more attention. Fortunately, just in the past five years there has begun to develop a body of serious, significant research on the evolution of human microbial pathogens. This newly emerging field of research has been termed "Darwinian medicine," and one of the most intriguing, promising, and readable studies in the field is published recently by Paul Ewald, evolutionary biologist at Amherst, under the title *The Evolution of Infectious Disease.* Marc Lappé, another writer in the field of Darwinian medicine, is also concerned about the possible evolution of HIV toward increased virulence. "The present evolutionary situation is anything but reassuring," he says.

> As the HIV-positive population burgeons toward 30 million, the opportunity for still greater evolutionary drift and change in the viruses associated with this disease increase accordingly. A vast reservoir of human hosts now provides a living evolutionary laboratory for a virus that knows no bounds.[16]

Whether HIV will tend to mutate toward increased virulence or toward decreased virulence, however, is still an open question. Some optimistic thinkers are hoping that the virus will mutate toward a more stable commensalism with its human hosts, but whether this will happen or not (at present, it looks rather unlikely) is an issue that will not be decided in this book. Instead we will move now to the issue on which this book focuses its attention, the question of finding an effective preventive vaccine.

3.4 A PREVENTIVE VACCINE?

The World Health Organization announced on May 8, 1980 that smallpox, a viral disease, had been completely eliminated from the earth.[17]

> The world and all its peoples have won freedom from smallpox, which was a most devastating disease sweeping in epidemic form through many countries since earliest times, leaving death, blindness, and disfigurement in its wake and which only a decade ago was rampant in Africa, Asia, and South America.[18]

This enormous feat was accomplished not by finding a cure but by finding a preventive vaccine and distributing it worldwide. Polio, another viral disease, has been largely erased from developed nations. WHO, in fact, announced in September of 1994 that polio had been completely eliminated from the Western hemisphere, and that polio was expected to be entirely eliminated from all nations by the year 2000. If that effort succeeds it will be due not to a cure but to a vaccine. Measles, mumps, rubella, diphtheria, and whooping cough, at least in the US and some other industrialized nations, are more or less under control, and in some countries have been eliminated, all due to vaccines.[19] The most successful strategy we have developed for fighting viral diseases has been to develop a preventive vaccine, and we have developed a number of them. In fact it has been said that in the area of general human health as a whole, the discovery and development of preventive vaccines has been the most significant medical development in our entire history. One historian of medicine has written that, "with the exception of safe water, no other modality, not even antibiotics, has had such a major effect on mortality reduction".[20]

Preventing a disease with a vaccine is inherently more effective than curing a disease with antibiotics or chemicals, for four reasons: a) because a preventive modality eliminates the sufferings of sickness altogether, whereas a curative modality only shortens those sufferings (which, of course, is extremely valuable for those who have already contracted the disease). b) A preventive modality also reduces the pathogen's pool of reproduction, since prevention actually stops the pathogen from finding another host; so in addition to preventing infection in the individual, it also reduces the likelihood of transmission to other hosts in the human population. c) This in turn has the additional advantage of reducing the pathogen's opportunities for mutation toward increased virulence (as we have seen above). And, finally, d) prevention is better than cure because prevention modalities, by their nature, strengthen our innate resistance mechanisms, rather than weaken them. Treatment with modern antibiotic and chemical therapies can often weaken our innate resistance to invading microbes, thereby making us ultimately more vulnerable than we were before we were treated.[21]

Ben Franklin was right when he had Poor Richard remind us that an ounce of prevention is worth a pound of cure.

A successful vaccine protection strategy against a human disease requires several things. It requires that we have a vaccine a) that is relatively effective in protecting people against the disease, b) that is easily transported and stored, c) that is resistant to a wide range of temperature change, d) that can be easily administered, and e) that requires only two or three administrations, perhaps four at most. We also want a vaccine f) that can be produced in high quantities, g) at low cost, and h) that can be distributed world wide. We can then administer the vaccine to virtually everyone in the population, or at least to everyone in the population who might be at some risk of becoming infected.

Vaccines with characteristics such as these, if they are efficacious in a large percentage of those vaccinated, both prevent sickness in the individual vaccinees, and also minimize the spread of the sickness in the human community. The virus then fails to catch hold (or fails to maintain its hold) in the population, for lack of immuno-innocent hosts, and dies out. The human hosts win and the viral parasites lose.

The question is: will it be possible to develop such a vaccine for the human immunodeficiency virus?

NOTES

1. Mauro Schecter, AIDS program Director at a university hospital in Rio de Janeiro. *New York Times,* 25 January 1993.
2. "Prevention is better than cure. Our victory over most infectious diseases owes more to vaccination than it does to drugs." M. D. Grmek MD, PhD. *History of AIDS: Emergence and Origin of a Modern Pandemic.* Trans. Maulitz, Russell, and Duffin, Jacalyn (Princeton, NJ: Princeton University Press, 1990) 279+xii., p 186.
3. J. Lederberg, "Pandemic as Natural Evolutionary Phenomenon," in A. Mack, ed. *In Time of Plague: The History and Social Consequences of Lethal Epidemic Disease* (New York: New York University Press, 1991) 206+xii., pp 29–30.
4. L. M. Simons. "AIDS cure impossible this century, predicts co-discoverer of virus." *The Seattle Times* 8 August 1994.

5. "HIV has demonstrated an ability to evolve resistance to virtually every drug that has been used against it." P. Ewald. *The Evolution of Infectious Disease* (Oxford University Press, 1994), p 170.
6. J. Mann, D. Tarantola and T. Netter, eds. *AIDS in the World* (Cambridge, MA: Harvard University Press, 1992) 1037+xvi., p 33.
7. In a chapter on non infectious immunosuppressive agents, Robert Root-Bernstein makes it clear that the overuse of antibiotics, for example, has been shown to cause temporary immunosuppression:

   It is certainly well established that most antibiotics can cause immune suppression when used in acute, high doses or at moderate doses taken over long periods of time. Many reports were published during the 1950s that high doses of penicillin compounds often resulted in opportunistic infections with various fungi and yeasts, such as Candida albicans . Chloramphenicol reduced both humoral and cell-mediated immunity to such an extent that foreign tissue graft survival was demonstrable. Tetracycline, streptomycin, kanamycin, gentamycin, and neomycin are immunosuppressive. Cefotaxime, anikacin, mezlocilin, piperacillin, and clindamycin have been described as 'immunomodulatory.' Specific inhibitory effects have been demonstrated on cell-mediated immunity for many of these antibiotics, suggesting T cell-mediated mechanisms. It is thought that some of the antibiotics depress immune function by tying up zinc, selenium, calcium, and other minerals necessary for cell division. R. Root-Bernstein. *Rethinking AIDS: The Tragic Cost of Premature Consensus* (New York, NY: The Free Press, Macmillan, 1993) 512+xv. pp 132–33. (When you check Root-Bernstein's citations for these data, you will see that they come from studies published in reputable journals like *Surgery* and *Lancet*, as well as a work published by Elsevier, in Amsterdam, titled "Immunotoxicology of Drugs and Chemicals".)

8. "A large proportion of women in Africa cannot reduce their risk of HIV infection because they already are monogamous and lack the autonomy to introduce condoms or other preventive measures into sexual interactions. . . .

   Progress in the control of HIV/AIDS in women and children in Africa is unlikely without improvement in the education, employment opportunities, and social status of women, which should be a policy objective for better health." K. M. De Cock MD, MRCP, DTM&H, et al., "The Public Health Implications of AIDS Research in Africa", *JAMA*, 272, 6.10 August (1994) 481–86., p 484.
9. "While acknowledging that he was calling for an effort to 'transform society to deal with AIDS,' Mann insisted that AIDS campaigners need not use the language of human rights to push for these changes because it is in the economic interest of nations to increase the productivity of their populations and lower the costs of caring for the sick." C. A. Radin. "AIDS fight portrayed as a failure; Prevention, education efforts fall short, global specialist says." *The Boston Globe* 10 August 1994. 1.

10. "The impact of conflict, social unrest, and population movement in developing countries on public health, including HIV/AIDS, merits much more attention." K. M. De Cock MD, MRCP, DTM&H, et al., "The Public Health Implications of AIDS Research in Africa", *JAMA*, 272, 6.10 August (1994) 481–86., p 482.
11. B. D. Schoub. *AIDS & HIV in Perspective* (New York, NY: Cambridge University Press, 1994) 268+xx., pp 245–46.
12. *Ibid.*
13. D. A. Feldman, ed. *Global AIDS Policy* (Westport, CT: Bergin & Garvey, 1994) 250+x., p 237.
14. The authors continue: "Nevertheless, many stable commensalisms and mutualistic symbioses have indeed evolved, culminating in the incorporation of mitochondria and chloroplasts as essential constituents of animal and plant cells." Cf. L. Margulis, *Symbiosis in Cell Evolution* (San Francisco: Freeman, 1982). Joshua Lederberg, "Pandemic as Natural Evolutionary Phenomenon," in, A. Mack, ed. *In Time of Plague: The History and Social Consequences of Lethal Epidemic Disease* (New York: New York University Press, 1991) 206+xii. pp 37–38.

    Cf. also the well-developed arguments supporting this conclusion in P. Ewald. *The Evolution of Infectious Disease* (Oxford University Press, 1994).
15. Joshua Lederberg, "Pandemic as Natural Evolutionary Phenomenon," in A. Mack, ed. *In Time of Plague: The History and Social Consequences of Lethal Epidemic Disease* (New York: New York University Press, 1991) 206+xii., pp 35–36.
16. M. Lappé. *Evolutionary Medicine: Rethinking the Origins of Disease* (San Francisco, CA: Sierra Club Books, 1994) 255+xii., p 135.
17. *Encyclopedia Britannica*, 1986.

    The eradication program "began with a proposal by Victor Zhdanov . . . Vice Minister of Health for the Soviet Union. It was the first serious statement by anyone [since Edward Jenner first believed in the idea] that we could even do this," said Donald A. Henderson, former director of the smallpox eradication program. C. Siebert. "Smallpox is Dead, Long Live Smallpox." *The New York Times Magazine* 21 August 1994, section 6, 31–55.

    The first person who seriously suggested that the disease of smallpox could actually be eliminated from the earth was indeed Edward Jenner, the discoverer and developer of the cowpox vaccine against smallpox.

    It is also intriguing to note that just as smallpox was eradicated from the earth, the first cases of severe acquired immunodeficiency were getting ready to be noticed by the Centers for Disease Control and Prevention in Atlanta, an organization that had also been a major player in the smallpox eradication program (SEP).
18. Quoted in L. Garrett. *The Coming Plague: Newly Emerging Diseases in a World Out of Balance* (New York, NY: Farrar, Straus and Giroux, 1994) 750+xiv, p 47.
19. D. Hodel and AIDS Action Foundation Working Group. *HIV Preventive Vaccines: Social, Ethical, and Political Considerations* (AIDS Action

Foundation, Office of AIDS Research, National Institutes of Health, 1994), p 2. See also B. D. Schoub. *AIDS & HIV in Perspective* (New York, NY: Cambridge University Press, 1994) 268+xx., p 183.
20. S. L. Plotkin and S. A. Plotkin. "A Short History of Vaccination." Trans. *Vaccines.* Eds. Stanley A. Plotkin and Edward A. Mortimer. second ed. (Philadelphia, PA: W.B. Saunders Co, 1994) 1–11, p 1.
21. M. Lappé. *Evolutionary Medicine: Rethinking the Origins of Disease* (San Francisco, CA: Sierra Club Books, 1994) 255+xii., p 212.

4 Is a Vaccine Possible?

Or, more precisely, the question is: if the economic disincentives can be overcome, will it be possible to develop such a vaccine for the human immunodeficiency virus? The vaccine question needs to be phrased thus because economic disincentives may present serious obstacles to vaccine development.

4.1 ECONOMIC DISINCENTIVES

Normal market forces are not favorable for enticing private pharmaceutical companies to commit themselves and their resources to the development of vaccines, and particularly not to the development of HIV vaccines. The expenses entailed by such research will be extremely high, the legal liabilities will be considerable, the probable financial return may be small, and the possibility of complete failure in the research is substantial.

4.1.1 Costs

Costs entailed by development and eventual testing of candidate HIV vaccines will probably be in the many hundreds of millions of dollars, and those dollars would probably be invested with anticipation of no great probability of success. Genentech Corporation in San Francisco, for example,

> has invested $150 million in AIDS research and has not been able to bring a single product to market, according to G. Kirk Raab, Genentech's president and chief executive officer. Raab says that unless [we] come up with something that looks much more promising than rgp120 [recombinant gp120 subunit vaccine], the company is not likely to continue to invest in AIDS vaccine research.[1]

4.1.2 Legal liabilities

Furthermore, the legal liabilities – i.e., the potential for being sued by persons or groups who feel they have been harmed by a vaccine – could be enormous, perhaps also ranging into the hundreds of millions of dollars. Historically, these potential vaccine-associated liabilities have been enough of a threat to discourage most pharmaceutical companies from making serious investments in vaccine research. In the US, some congressionally mandated measures have been developed to minimize these liabilities in recent years, but HIV vaccine researchers still feel they need to be fiscally cautious.

4.1.3 Financial return

In addition, the possible financial return on even a fairly successful vaccine is not expected to be great, especially if the primary markets for the vaccines would be in developing nations, where the setting of higher prices for vaccines would probably be viewed as unnecessarily (and unethically) exploitative.

In other words, the costs are expected to be high, the legal liabilities are expected to be severe, and the financial returns are expected to be modest. These are not the sort of market forces that would normally induce a company to commit itself to investing in vaccine research.[2]

Supposing, however, that some solutions to these economic disincentives can be found (and I believe that economically creative solutions will eventually emerge), there is still serious question as to whether it will be possible to develop a successful HIV vaccine. For one thing, the scientific challenges are formidable.

4.2 SCIENTIFIC CHALLENGES

Whether it will be scientifically possible to develop a preventive vaccine for HIV is, as yet, an unanswered question, but, since a vaccine would be such a gargantuan boon for humanity, there is a great deal of work being done around the world to develop such a vaccine. In 1984, when the virus was first isolated and the world was told – by Robert Gallo in the United States and Luc Montagnier in Paris – that we had now discovered the infectious agent that causes AIDS, public health officials and scientists alike were confident that a vaccine could not be far away. On Monday, April 23, 1984, the day that the discovery of "the AIDS virus" was announced, US Health and Human Services Secretary Margaret Heckler "took to the podium . . . to assert that a blood test would be available in six months and a vaccine would be tested in two years".[3] Her optimism turned out to be a bit hasty.

In the intervening twelve years hopes for a vaccine have been raised and then dashed several times, until some researchers have become frankly skeptical that there will ever be a vaccine for this virus.

Dr William Haseltine, for example, Chief of the Division of Retrovirology at the Dana-Farber Cancer Institute in Boston, is highly skeptical about the hope for vaccine successes. Speaking at the 1993 annual meeting of the American Association for the Advancement of Science, he said, "Do you want to know my guess for the chance that any of these vaccines that we're trying now will work? Zero." He said, moreover, that much AIDS research is "a mistake in the allocation of resources," because the chances of developing an effective vaccine are so small.[4]

This skepticism is, in many respects, entirely warranted. In this chapter and the next three chapters I will explain why this skepticism is warranted, and yet why vaccine research will continue to be pursued in the hope that it may yield some significant prevention for HIV infection. Drs José Esparza, William Heyward, and Saladin Osmanov, Directors of the effort for HIV vaccine development at WHO in Geneva, are certainly some of the most knowledgeable specialists in the world in the area of HIV vaccine research. The AIDS Vaccine Development Unit at WHO is presently spearheading a major new initiative for HIV vaccine development, in collaboration with the pharmaceutical industry. WHO wants to determine now, or at least soon, whether a vaccine for HIV is indeed possible. Drs Esparza, Heyward, and Osmanov are quite hopeful that an HIV vaccine will eventually be developed, despite the skepticism of some researchers.

The skepticism springs from an understanding of a) the nature of the human immunodeficiency virus itself and b) the nature of the way vaccines work. So we need to take a brief side trip to elucidate one or two key characteristics of the virus, and to review how the immune system works. (Readers who are fully familiar with HIV and who are also familiar with the workings of the human immune system, may choose to skip ahead to Chapter 8, the discussion of human trials.)

NOTES

1. *Los Angeles Times*, 9 August 1994, part A, p 1.
2. Consider:

   [P]reventive vaccines . . . sell at low prices, are not very profitable, and often are not used – even when supplied free of charge. While the economic incentives are virtually non-existent, the risks associated with the many unknown facets of HIV and with testing candidate vaccines are great. . . . Steps must be taken to remove the barriers that deter biopharmaceutical firms from pursuing vaccines. D. P. Francis. "A Private-Sector AIDS Vaccine? Don't Hold Your Breath." *Washington Post* 19 July 1994. A17.

   These are the very reasons that we may be more likely to see successful HIV vaccine research come out of government sponsored laboratories than out of private sector research laboratories.
3. J. Kinsella. *Covering the Plague: AIDS and the American Media* (New Brunswick, NJ: Rutgers University Press, 1989) 299+x., p 84.
4. M. F. Goldsmith, "For AIDS Treatment, Vaccines, Now Think Genes", *JAMA*, 269, 17. 5 May (1993) 2189–90, p 2189.

   Consider also Paul Ewald's statement: "[D]eveloping a safe and effective AIDS vaccine will be one of the most formidable challenges ever assigned to health sciences, and the foreseeable difficulties translate into millions of deaths from AIDS before a vaccine that is even moderately effective will be put into use." P. Ewald. *The Evolution of Infectious Disease* (Oxford University Press, 1994), p 177.

   Consider also Wayne Koff's statement about all the present generation of candidate HIV vaccines: "None of these products will likely enter efficacy trials either in the United States or elsewhere, because of their inability in phase I trials to induce or maintain the levels of immune responses likely to be effective against HIV." Also: "Resources should no longer be targeted to first generation vaccines that have little or no potential for success." W. C. Koff, "The Next Steps Toward a Global AIDS Vaccine", *Science*, 266.25 November (1994) 1335–37, pp 1336, 1337.

5 The Human Immunodeficiency Virus

5.1 ETIOLOGICITY

By far the greatest bulk of opinion in the intelligent AIDS research community is that HIV is the cause, the etiologic agent, for AIDS. I should probably not refer to their belief as "opinion," and should not even refer to it as "belief," since it is based on an enormous amount of thought and research. But there is a small number of intelligent persons, such as Robert Root-Bernstein and others, who dissent from this view, some of whom have quite impressive credentials. (There are also, as always, a number of not so thoughtful dissenters.) This small number of renegade researchers – even though many of them disagree even among themselves[1] – continues to question how certain we should be that HIV is the etiologic agent for AIDS. They are still actively debating the issue, presenting data, and pursuing the argument, and their efforts must not be minimized. Still, most AIDS researchers feel that the evidence is compelling that HIV does cause AIDS. A recent issue of *Science* reported on the journal's latest, quite thorough, three-month investigation of the arguments and evidence for this minority thesis, and still concluded that the evidence supporting the HIV-causes-AIDS thesis was very compelling.[2]

Unfortunately, however, an important ingredient has been missing from the debate: there has been very little discussion of what *standard* should be used to determine whether an agent is etiologic for a certain disease. I think the issue of what standard should be used for determining etiologicity is an issue that deserves much more attention, and I have seen very little discussion of it. Most authors repeat Robert Koch's four postulates in one form or another, but then acknowledge that his postulates should be taken as guidelines only, and not as absolutes.

Very briefly, Koch's four postulates for determining that a given microbe is etiologic for a given disease are, in rough form, the following: a) That unique microbe must be found present in all cases of the disease. b) That unique microbe must be able to be taken from the host and isolated in a pure culture. c) Inoculations of that cultured microbe into animal hosts must then produce in those hosts the identical disease. d) That unique microbe must then be able to be taken from the new hosts and again isolated in pure culture. In other words, if you find the exact same microbe in all cases of a disease, if you are able to culture that microbe and inject it into another host so that that host too gets the same disease, and then if you are able to culture that microbe out of all the newly diseased hosts, then at that point you can safely say that that microbe is indeed etiologic for that particular disease. That bug causes that disease.

Researchers on both sides of the argument acknowledge, however, that these postulates were devised in the context of Koch's research on bacteria, and therefore may have only passing relevance to research on viruses. It is, after all, a much more difficult matter to isolate viruses than it is to culture bacteria. Therefore, it may be that these criteria simply do not apply to research involving viral diseases. Furthermore, the critics point out, Koch suggested those four postulates as guidelines only and not as rigid standards of absolute necessity. (The recent report in *Science,* however, is not so quick to concede that HIV does not satisfy Koch's postulates; it presents recent evidence to support the claim that HIV does indeed satisfy Koch's postulates, and therefore does meet this rather high standard of being etiologic for AIDS.[3])

Sadly, I have seen little discussion of any other possible standards of etiologicity. Certainly, Robert Heubner's (past chief of the Laboratory of RNA Tumor Viruses at the National Cancer Institute in Bethesda, Maryland) eight postulates deserve serious consideration. Without going into any of the details of his postulates, they are at least a more precise set of criteria, and they have been devised specifically to determine etiologicity in research with viruses. Root-Bernstein discusses these postulates at length (as well as some other sets of criteria by Tom Rivers, Robert Gallo and others) but then Root-Bernstein concludes that none of these standards adequately applies to HIV.

> Neither Heubner's nor Rivers's criteria have been addressed by HIV proponents. Either they do not know them, or they know that HIV does not satisfy them any more than it satisfies Koch's postulates. . . . In short, HIV does not satisfy any of the etiologic criteria that existed prior to its discovery, and the etiologic criteria that have been developed since [such as Robert Gallo's] are all logically flawed.[4]

The debate about whether HIV is etiologic for AIDS is significant in the context of this book, of course, because all of the vaccines presently under development are vaccines against HIV, which most researchers are convinced is a virtually necessary (though perhaps not sufficient) condition for acquiring AIDS. If HIV is not a necessary condition for developing AIDS, then the vaccines against HIV now under development would not have the significance researchers presently believe them to have.

This debate about whether HIV is the cause of AIDS generated a great deal of heat during 1993 and 1994 in a sort of standoff between the highly respected journal *Nature*, and a British newspaper, *The Sunday Times*. I quote from an editorial in *Nature*, December 9, 1993:

> [T]he causation of AIDS has been a profound disappointment to the research community. Almost ten years have passed since HIV was first recognized, but the evidence that it causes AIDS is still epidemiological. The mechanism of the pathogenesis of the disease has not yet been uncovered (although parts of Duesberg's 'challenge' have been met), so that the evidence necessarily seems circumstantial. But the vast majority of the evidence is consistent with the view that HIV is a cause (and probably a sufficient cause) of AIDS. How, in these circumstances, can *The Sunday Times* so consistently assert the opposite?[5]

The thrust of this editorial is clearly in support of the "HIV causes AIDS" thesis, and thus it represents the bulk of opinion in the intelligent AIDS research community. The first three sentences, however, do seem to allow some room for leaving the question open.

A very important contribution to this dialog is the lengthy, serious, booklength argument by Robert Root-Bernstein that argues that HIV may play a role other than simply being a sufficient or necessary condition for the development of AIDS. His argument, I hope, will provoke a detailed response from the research community.[6]

However, this debate must be tabled for now, important as it is, and the final decision on its outcome left to the investigations of competent virologists and epidemiologists. But, since current AIDS vaccine research is based on the conviction that HIV is at least a necessary condition for AIDS, it will be best for now to go with the conviction of most serious researchers, and to assume, or at least to stipulate (in the legal sense), that HIV is probably a necessary condition for all, or virtually all, cases of AIDS.[7]

If this is the case, then it would indeed make a great deal of sense to look for a preventive vaccine that would protect against HIV.

5.2 ALIVE?

What are some of the characteristics of this Human Immunodeficiency Virus?

In the first place, as a virus it inhabits a kind of gray zone at the edge of life,[8] situated somewhere between life and non-life. Most microbiology textbooks refer to viruses as particles which are no more than combinations of nucleic acids and protein molecules. This makes them merely clusters of chemicals, particles of matter that have only the kind of simplistic actions and reactions that other chemicals have. Viruses, these texts point out, have few if any characteristics of things that are alive, so they should not be called living things. Other microbiology textbooks, however, refer to viruses as microbes, or even as microorganisms, implying that they are in some way alive, even if only in a most elemental way. Which is the case? Is a virus alive or not alive? The truth is that this is probably more a lexical question about the definition of "life," and about what characteristics a being must have before it can be termed "living," than it is a substantive question to be answered by microbiologists. Consider, for example, the following remarks by Arnold Levine, Chair of the Department of Molecular Biology at Princeton and editor-in-chief of the *Journal of Virology*.

> Viruses, as we have seen, can program their own replication within the confines of a cell. They have a plan, satisfying Aristotle's definition of life, encoded in the format of all living things. And, like other living things, viruses evolve and respond to environmental changes. Whether this describes the simplest of living forms or an extraordinarily complex combination of nucleic acids and proteins that are merely chemicals depends upon one's view of life.[9]

This definitional question does not need to be conclusively answered here, but since I commonly see viruses referred to as "microorganisms," even in the scientific literature, I will also feel free to so refer to them here.

5.3 VIROLOGY AND MUTABILITY

More relevant to our purposes, however, is the fact that HIV is a retrovirus, i.e., an RNA based virus rather than a DNA based virus, and thus is one of the few "living" things that has no DNA code in it. HIV, which in the context of this book means primarily HIV-1 – HIV-1 is presently responsible for more than 90 per cent of the HIV infections in the world, with HIV-2 being responsible for the other nine to ten per cent[10] – attacks one of the chief cells in the immune system. But even more importantly than that, and partly as a result of its being a retrovirus, it is an especially mutable virus. Every time it enters a human cell it takes over the reproductive machinery within the cell and turns that machinery to its own reproductive purposes. The cell then reproduces thousands, even hundreds of thousands, of new virions, virtual copies of the parent virus. These daughter virus particles (as virologists refer to them) then exit the cell, and each one seeks out another cell to infect and take over, again using that cell's machinery to replicate virtual copies of itself. The key word here is "virtual". The daughter virus particles are almost exact replications of the parent virus, but the replicating machinery often makes small mistakes, and hence the new generation of viruses has some degree of variation, or mutation, from the original virus. Each generation of HIV (from each infected human cell) contains some percentage of variations, or mutations, from the parent virus, and HIV has much more than its proper share of such variations.[11] In fact, it is the most mutable virus known.[12] Until discovery of this virus, it was commonly said that the influenza virus was the most mutable virus known, because each generation changed its coat to some degree. Now, as Robert Gallo has reported, every single generation of HIV has been shown to be different in some degree.

> Genetic diversity, or the production of HIV variants, is a major problem in vaccine development. In 1988, Robert Gallo . . . reported that *every* HIV isolate has been different. Even sequential HIV isolates from the same patient differ and demonstrate different susceptibilities to a standard neutralizing antibody. . . . [A] report from Gallo's laboratory [states] that even a *single amino acid* change in the HIV envelope can result in a virus that resists the same neutralization antibodies that had previously neutralized parent HIV. Further, it has been reported that at least 25% of the amino acids in HIV envelope protein are subject to change at any time during the production of HIV.[13]

HIV's high mutation rate works very much to its advantage and, hence, to our disadvantage as its hosts. Mutability (or variability), in general, works to the advantage of a species, particularly if the species inhabits a relatively dynamic environment. Lack of variability, on the other hand, is not to a species' advantage, because when its environment changes and the species does not change to adapt to the new environment, then the species suffers. This principle of evolutionary ecology works to the great advantage of all microorganisms that are mutable, particularly those microorganisms that want to live in an environment as complex and dynamic as the human body and its immune system. The high variability of these microorganisms makes it possible for them to mutate their way around – i.e., become resistant to – antibiotic and antiviral medications. This is the case with the new drug-resistant strains of *M. tuberculosis,* with drug-resistant forms of malaria parasites, and with a variety of other, newly-resistant human pathogens.

One problem with a virus such as HIV that has a rapid replication and mutation rate, and hence such a high degree of variability, is that the immune system is then constantly challenged by new forms of the virus, which our cells must then track down, recognize, and mount a new defense against. The defenses of the immune system, after all, are not generic defenses but are *specific* defenses, against *this* specific invader. So each time there is a new invader, or a viral mutant that looks like a new invader, a new defense must be mounted. The new defense, of course, always takes some finite amount of time to develop. This presents an enormous challenge to the immune system. It also presents an enormous challenge to vaccine researchers, because each vaccine they develop is also a vaccine against a specific invader which has a specific form. "To appreciate the difficulty in generating an AIDS vaccine," explains Paul Ewald

> consider the influenza virus, which has a mutation rate slightly less than that of HIV. . . . [T]hese new flu strains can be dealt with effectively if surveillance is diligent and resources are ready. One need only identify the epidemic type, grow it, kill it, and circulate it as a vaccine to combat the epidemic. . . . [But] unlike the influenza virus, HIV has no "AIDS season." Trying to control HIV's spread with a vaccine is like trying to control all of the flu epidemics of the next century at once with a single flu vaccine.[14]

Hence, although we are able to develop and distribute new vaccines against the highly mutable flu virus every year, the challenge to do the same against HIV, which has such an immense variety of wild strains, is almost impossible. The skeptics think it *is* impossible.

NOTES

1. I monitor a discussion group/listserve on the internet, called "Rethinking AIDS," which is composed of persons who disagree with the HIV-causes-AIDS hypothesis. Some of their discussion is intriguing, though highly contentious, and there is not as much agreement among their ranks as they might like. Most of them, however, do support the hypotheses of Peter Duesberg. See P. Duesberg, *Inventing the AIDS Virus*, (Washington, DC: Regnery, 1996) 722.
2. J. Cohen, "The Duesberg Phenomenon", *Science*, 266.9 December (1994) 1642–49, p 1642.
3. *Ibid.*, p 1647.
4. R. Root-Bernstein. *Rethinking AIDS: The Tragic Cost of Premature Consensus* (New York, NY: The Free Press, Macmillan, 1993) 512+xv, p 100.
5. Editor, "Editorial", Nature, 366, 6455.9 December (1993) 493–94.
6. R. Root-Bernstein. *Rethinking AIDS: The Tragic Cost of Premature Consensus.* (New York, NY: The Free Press, Macmillan, 1993) 512+xv.
7. Having said that, however, critics of the HIV-causes-AIDS thesis should probably also be aware of the following historical detail:

   It is, of course, true that the most efficient technique for finding a successful vaccine against a given disease is to first identify the pathogen that causes the disease, and then to develop a vaccine that is directed specifically against that pathogen. That is the method which scientific medicine has used for the development of vaccines for the past 100 years, and it has been a successful method.

   Still, it should be remembered that the first vaccine that was ever developed by the method of scientific testing (and in many ways the most successful vaccine we have developed so far), viz., the vaccine against smallpox, was developed (by Edward Jenner in the 18th century) in total ignorance of the causal agent for smallpox. And worse than that, the successful discovery of that vaccine also emerged in total ignorance of the mechanisms of pathogenesis that operated to produce smallpox disease in a person. Yet, in spite of such ignorances, a highly successful vaccine was developed against one of the worst infectious diseases ever to affect human beings. This historical reminder may give some substance to the hopes of those who still believe it will be possible to develop a vaccine for protection against HIV and/or AIDS.

   See my book, *Jenner on Trial: An Ethical Examination of Vaccine Research in the Age of Smallpox and the Age of AIDS.* See also G. L. Ada, "Modern Vaccines," *The Lancet*, 335, March 3 (1990) 523–26, p 523.
8. See E. B. Wilson. *At the Edge of Life: an introduction to viruses.* NIH Publication 80–433 (Washington DC: US Department of Health and Human Services, Government Printing Office, 1980) 75.
9. A. J. Levine. *Viruses* (New York, NY: Scientific American Library, 1992) 241+xii, p 22.
10. W. C. Koff, "The Next Steps Toward a Global AIDS Vaccine", *Science*, 266.25 November (1994) 1335–37, p 1337.

11. HIV is so mutable that there may be numerous different "quasi-species" within one individual host." B. D. Schoub. *AIDS & HIV in Perspective* (New York, NY: Cambridge University Press, 1994) 268+xx, p 65.
12. Cf. three recent books on the emerging field of Darwinian medicine: Ewald, Paul, *The Evolution of Infectious Disease* (Oxford University Press, 1994), M. Lappé, *Evolutionary Medicine: Rethinking the Origins of Disease* (San Francisco, CA: Sierra Club Books, 1994) 255+xii; and Fisher, Jeffrey A., *The Plague Makers: How We are Creating Catastrophic New Epidemics – and What We Must Do to Avert Them* (New York: Simon & Schuster, 1994) 256.
13. Ada, George. "Prospects for a Vaccine Against HIV." *Nature* 339 (1989): 331–32, as quoted in Stine, Gerald. *Acquired Immune Deficiency Syndrome: Biological, Medical, Social and Legal Issues.* First ed. Englewood Cliffs (NJ 07632: Prentice Hall, 1993) 462+xxxii, 214.

    Ewald believes that part of the explanation for the high variability of HIV may be that "HIV's reverse transcriptase tends to generate mutations at greater rates than the reverse transcriptases of other retroviruses" P. Ewald. *The Evolution of Infectious Disease* (Oxford University Press, 1994) p 153. Retroviruses generate mutations at a much greater rate than regular DNA viruses.
14. P. Ewald. *The Evolution of Infectious Disease* (Oxford University Press, 1994) p 175.

6 How the Immune System Works

The primary function of the immune system, to say it in the most elemental (and oversimplified, but not altogether untrue) terms, is to distinguish between what is self and what is non-self, and then to eliminate the non-self. Thus, whenever a non-self substance breaks the normal skin and membrane barriers of the body and gets "inside the walls," the immune system shifts into gear to meet the challenge. If the invader is a microbe, such as a bacterium or virus, macrophage cells seek it out, surround it, and try to ingest and absorb it. They then transport portions of it over to another cell in the system, the T4 cell, the cell that oversees and regulates the entire cellular and humoral immune response, and present the surface of that invader to the surface of the T4 cell for recognition. "See what I have here?" it seems to say. "Well, there are more out there just like this one, and they have the same coat this one has. Let's gear up for them, train our troops to recognize them, and fight them off. What say? Should we get to battle stations?"[1]

Thus begins the buildup to fight against this specific invader with this specific coat. The T4 cell starts to instruct other cells, B cells, T8 cells, CTL cells, and others, to start multiplying their numbers and performing their necessary functions. Interleukins, chemical messengers that carry instructions from one cell to another, are manufactured and secreted. Antibodies are concocted to fit the surface molecules of the invader, are manufactured by the billions, and are sent out into the bloodstream to affix themselves to the surface of every invader found. Many preparations are made for the battle, and these preparations take some finite amount of time to adequately be accomplished. In the meantime, the invaders are invading, are multiplying their own forces, and are beginning to have their toxic effect on the body (assuming that the invading microorganism is pathogenic to some extent). They are making the body sick. If, for example, the invading microbe is a rhinovirus, the human being begins to feel a cold coming on, begins to feel headachey, run down, tired, and maybe feels a fever developing. As the microbes multiply during the next hours or days, and as the immune system is building up its defenses, the human being is experiencing the pathogenic effects of the invader.

It will probably be several days before the forces of the immune system are able to overcome the forces of the invading rhinovirus, and the body can get the bug under control. After the battle is won by the immune system and the microbes are finally conquered, then the immune system cells can rest from their work, can stand down, relax, and go back to semi-dormancy. But – and the "but" here is enormously significant – now they remember (by means of T and B memory cells) exactly how they defeated that invader, so that next time they can defeat it much more rapidly. The next time they encounter that same invader, and its particular bag of tricks, they will be ready to fight it in full force almost immediately. They will not suffer from that very costly time delay to ready their defenses. They can start the battle at once and conquer the invaders before they have a chance to multiply and do their pathogenic work. In fact, the immune system cells will probably conquer the invaders before the human being in which all this is happening even knows there has been an invasion. The body will not even get sick the second time.

And that is exactly how and why vaccines work.

NOTES

1. Xenophobic as the "self/other" metaphor might sound to some readers, and as seemingly paranoid as the "invader/self-defense/battle" metaphors might sound to some pacifists, it is, nonetheless, a way of understanding the immune system that has become the standard in immunology textbooks, and probably will continue to be the standard for some time, because this form of "immunosemiotics" works so effectively in describing the variety of actual mechanisms that make up the immune system.

Nevertheless, for an attempt to view the immune system using metaphors that are less military and less xenophobic, see the critique by anthropologist Emily Martin at Johns Hopkins. Her critique, though ultimately incomplete and unsatisfying in my opinion, is still intriguing and suggestive. E. Martin. *Flexible Bodies: Tracking Immunity in American Culture, from the Days of Polio to the Age of AIDS* (Boston: Beacon Press, 1994) 320+xxiv.

7 How Vaccines Work

Successful immunization methods for preventing smallpox were actually discovered in China, India and Africa more than a thousand years ago. "As early as the 10th century, the Chinese were taking the dried scabs of previous smallpox victims and blowing them up the nose of healthy people to ward off the disease."[1] One early Chinese medical text actually listed five different methods of inoculating persons against smallpox.

> (1) the nose plugged with powdered scabs laid on cotton wool, (2) powdered scabs blown into the nose, (3) the undergarments of an infected child put on a healthy child for several days, and (4) a piece of cotton smeared with the contents of a vesicle and stuffed into the nose. In addition, a century before Jenner, the Chinese used white cow fleas for smallpox prevention. The white cow fleas were ground into powder and made into pills, which presumably was the first attempt at an oral vaccine.[2]

In the fifth century BC, Thucydides' account of the Peloponnesian war between Athens and Sparta contains one of the first written accounts of the idea of natural immunity, that is, the idea that a person who contracts a disease once and who survives it, is then immune from contracting the disease again. Thucydides describes a terrible plague that struck Athens in 429 and 430 BC. His description sounds very much like an account of a smallpox epidemic, and includes the statement that "the same man was never attacked [by the same disease] twice". Therefore, says Thucydides, persons who recovered from an attack of the disease

> received not only the congratulations of others, but themselves also, in the elation of the moment, half entertained the vain hope that they were for the future safe from any disease whatsoever.[3]

They were not, of course, immune from all diseases, but they did seem to be immune from that particular one.

It was then later discovered that some other diseases also seemed to induce a natural immunity to further attacks of the disease. This then led to the notion of trying to artificially induce mild forms of disease in people, in hopes of immunizing them against future more virulent attacks of that disease. Jules Bordet, in his *Traite de l'immunite dans les Maladies Infectieuses,* in 1920, summarized the matter thus.

> Since a first attack, which strengthens the host, often provides valuable safeguards for the future, it must be considered desirable, on condition, of course, that it does not produce too much serious damage. Artificially putting the host into a state comparable to that in which it would be if it had been cured of a spontaneous attack of the particular illness is the object of active immunization or vaccination.[4]

This idea must doubtless have been the origin of the concept of artificial immunization.

In the early 1700s, a few travelers to the Near East, Africa and India brought word of artificial immunization practices back to Europe, particularly to England where it became a relatively common practice. Then, in 1796, Edward Jenner conducted experiments to determine whether inoculation with cowpox disease would produce immunity to smallpox disease.[5]

But whether the immunization procedures were done in 10th century China with powdered scabs, in late 18th century England with lancets, or in the late 20th century US with needles or sugar cubes (polio), the principles of vaccination are identical. When a body is vaccinated, immunized, variolated or inoculated (all of which words derive from different etymologies,[6] but mean approximately the same thing) that body is artificially introduced to a pathogen. Or, more precisely, a pathogen is introduced into that body. Or to be still more precise, some form of the pathogen (e.g., an attenuated form of the virus, a form that has been somehow artificially weakened), or some form of something very like the pathogen (as in using cowpox virus, for example, to inoculate against smallpox), or some fragmentary portion of the pathogen (e.g., using only the coat of the virus, minus the genetic material inside its core), or some artificially grown unit that looks like a fragmentary portion of the pathogen (e.g., a genetically engineered molecule which is identical to a molecule on the coat of the virus) is introduced into the body by injection, scarification, ingestion or suppository.

This constitutes the inoculation.

In some cases the body does get moderately sick from that inoculation, and sometimes it does not get sick at all. In either case, it mounts an immune response against that pathogen, and – most importantly – it remembers how a successful response was accomplished. The immune system is thus alerted, ready and charged, waiting for a time when it might see a real, wild variety of that pathogen trying to get in. When it does see such an invader, i.e., when it is "challenged" with a wild virus (or bacterium or whatever it was vaccinated against), it will be ready. It will be able to fight off that invading pathogen without the person's body ever feeling any sickness at all. The vaccine, you could say, "took". It worked. The person will not get sick from that pathogen for as long as the immune system memory cells remember that invader and that successful response.

That is how vaccines work.[7] They prepare a body for the battle, so that when the real wild virus comes along, the immune system will be able to a) recognize the virus by its coat, and b) fight it off before the pathogen can replicate itself in large enough numbers to cause disease. Vaccines, in other words, do not prevent initial infection with the invading virus; they prevent disease. Infection occurs, the immune system fights off the pathogenic invading microorganism, and disease does not occur.

But what does "fighting off the pathogen" mean? In the case of an invading virus it may mean either of two things. It may mean that a) the immune system is able to completely eliminate all the invading virus particles from the body, or it may mean only that b) the immune system is able to keep the invading viruses in check, and somehow under control. If the immune system does not completely eliminate the invading virus, then there remains the theoretical possibility that the virus particles which remain in the body could, at some future date, break free and again threaten to cause disease. (For a fuller discussion of possible modes of vaccine protection, see Chapter 9 below: Criteria of Effectiveness.)

The important key, however, is that before any immune response at all can happen, the invading wild virus must first of all be recognized by the immune system as the same virus that it was vaccinated against. If it is not so recognized, then the immune system does not mount a response, the invader's invasion succeeds, and the person gets the disease.

And that is the key problem that worries researchers and makes many of them skeptical that there will ever be a vaccine for HIV. For, as Robert Gallo has said, "every HIV isolate has been different". They are all wearing different coats. When the immune system is prepared for a virus that is wearing one coat, and is then challenged with a virus wearing a different coat, it does not respond in the way it was trained to respond. It has to make up another new response, and that will probably be an ultimately unsuccessful response. The person will get the disease.

7.1 CELL-ASSOCIATED TRANSMISSION

One additional problem that concerns researchers, and that makes some of them skeptical that there will ever be a successful HIV vaccine, is the problem of cell-associated transmission. HIV can be transmitted from one person to another either as viral particles floating freely in the bloodstream (or other tissues or fluids), or it can be transmitted from one person to another *within* certain cells. This is analogous to the way Agamemnon's warriors got inside the walls of Troy by hiding inside a large hollow wooden horse which was then wheeled into the city. If the virus is hiding inside the cells of an HIV-infected person, and some of those infected cells are transmitted to another person via one of the usual modes of transmission – sexual intercourse, needle-sharing or some other blood-borne path, for example – then the newly infected person's immune system would not be alerted to the presence of the viral invader in the same way it is alerted when the virus is floating free.[8] The virus would have successfully sneaked into the new host as a stowaway inside a cell. That virus, in fact, could continue to replicate itself by the thousands inside that cell or cells, and not be recognized by the new host's immune system until well after the virus had replicated itself enough times to insure a successful assault. This, in fact, is probably a common form of transmission of the virus from one host to another, and it causes a serious problem for vaccine protection. Paul Ewald explains:

> Compounding all of the problems associated with HIV's variability is the fact that HIV can infect susceptible people . . . without leaving infected cells. . . . Vaccines that are effective against free virus may have little effect on the progression of disease because HIV apparently often infects people within the disguising cloak of our cellular membranes; and infected cells may be far more effective than free virus at spreading infection. . . . The successes at vaccination are therefore only mildly encouraging.[9]

Complicating this problem is the likelihood that almost all sexual transmission is probably of the cell-associated type.[10] Since by far the most common mode of transmission of HIV in the world is sexual transmission (86 per cent),[11] this means that most HIV transmission in the world is of the cell-associated type. It is clear, therefore, that any vaccine that does not successfully address the difficulty of cell-associated transmission will not be a very successful vaccine.

These two problems alone, high replication and mutation rates of HIV, and cell-associated transmission, are what make many researchers skeptical of ever finding a successful vaccine against HIV.

But there are additional problems as well. One is that "the successes at vaccination" to which Ewald refers in the passage above are few and far between, and have occurred in animals rather than humans. Furthermore, they have been in animals that were vaccinated against simian immunodeficiency virus (SIV),[12] not against HIV. This raises the thorny issue of the "animal model," which every medical researcher sorely hopes to have for their research.

7.2 ANIMAL MODELS

If you do not have an animal that you can infect with the pathogen you are studying, then it is virtually impossible to do most medical research involving infectious agents. AIDS researchers, unfortunately, are not blessed with any very adequate animal model for their researches. They do have animals that can be infected with the human immunodeficiency virus, (chimpanzees) but the animals do not get sick from it. They do develop HIV antibodies, but for some reason they do not get AIDS.[13] So vaccinating them against HIV in order to prevent disease doesn't make any sense.[14] The animals don't get sick anyhow. An additional problem with chimps is that they are in short supply and are very expensive to maintain. So expensive in fact – they cost between $60,000 and $100,000 each to purchase – that there are only about 70 chimps in AIDS research in the entire US.[15]

Other animals (laboratory raised rhesus macaque monkeys) can be infected and caused to get sick and develop AIDS, but their AIDS is not caused by HIV. It is caused by SIV.[16] Consequently, much AIDS vaccine research is done with SIV models. SIV vaccines have sometimes yielded protection against disease in monkeys, but even in those cases, the protection occurred only when vaccinated monkeys were challenged (some months after the experimental vaccine was administered) with an SIV of the exact same (homologous) strain as the strain that the vaccine was modeled after. Those vaccines did not protect against any other wild strains of SIV. Any HIV vaccine that protected against only one strain of HIV would have very limited usefulness.

Another potentially promising animal model, announced in 1992 by scientists at the Washington Regional Primate Center in Seattle, is a colony of pigtail macaque monkeys which do seem to develop AIDS-like conditions when infected with HIV. The Seattle group is still hopeful about the success of this animal model, and so are some other researchers. Shortly after the 1992 announcement, there was a big run on the importation of pigtail macaques for US AIDS laboratories.

Not everyone feels so optimistic, however, about the pigtail macaque model. It has been found, for example, that

> in larger tests, pigtails have not gotten consistently sick or stayed that way. In some animals, the infection seems to be a passing thing. In many of the monkeys, antibodies against the virus show up and then seem to just start disappearing, as if the virus had made a feint and backed off. "I'm skeptical," admits [virologist Nick] Lerche. "It doesn't seem to be living up to the potential or hopes of that model. What I'm hearing now is yes, you can infect, but the infection is transient. . . . It doesn't seem any better than the chimp model."[17]

Even this hopeful animal model, it seems, may have some serious weaknesses. Actually, most animal models in medical research have some weaknesses; many drugs that are safe in humans are not safe in some animals, and vice versa. For example, penicillin is toxic in guinea pigs and hamsters, but not in most humans. Aspirin is toxic in cats and causes birth defects in mice and rats, but not in humans. Thalidomide, which causes severe birth defects in humans, causes no birth defects at all in at least 10 different strains of rats, nor "in 15 mouse strains, 11 rabbit breeds, 2 dog breeds, 3 hamster strains, and 8 other species of monkeys."[18] Almost no animal model in medical research is a fully adequate analog to human experience. For this reason, whatever we learn in laboratories and whatever we learn from tests in animals must be taken with a large grain of salt when we use those data to make predictions about what results to expect when we test the vaccine or drug in human subjects. The animal model may turn out to be a moderately accurate predictor of what to expect in human subjects, or it may turn out to be a quite inadequate predictor. In either case, at least with HIV candidate vaccines, we will not really know how good the animal model was until *after* we actually test the vaccine in human subjects. As Robert Levine says of animal models:

> Ordinarily, there is some background of experience derived from research on animals that will help predict with varying degrees of confidence what the risks might be to humans. However, it must be understood clearly that one never knows what the adverse (or, for that matter, beneficial) effects of any intervention in humans will be until the intervention has been tested adequately in humans.[19]

All these current problems with animal models for AIDS and HIV infection are, of course, subject to change. A successful animal model may in fact be developed at some point. Within the week previous to my writing this sentence, for example, *Science* reported the development of a possible baboon model for HIV-2 infection that may prove to be valuable.[20] Nevertheless, we need to be always mindful of the fundamental predictive limitations of relying very heavily on any animal model.

For all these reasons, many researchers have become skeptical about the possibility of ever developing a successful vaccine against HIV: the virus is too mutable, it can temporarily escape immune detection by intracellular transmission, and we do not yet have any very reliable or successful animal models that have given promising results. Paul Ewald expresses some of this skepticism when he compares our vaccine successes in the past to today's efforts:

> The success of vaccines against smallpox, yellow fever, whooping cough, and measles raised hopes that all pathogens could be controlled by vaccines. But as it turns out, some of the conquered pathogens were particularly oafish adversaries. A smallpox virus, for example, carried antigens that were also carried by virtually all other smallpox viruses as well as its taxonomic relative, the vaccinia virus [which causes cowpox], which is the virus used in the smallpox vaccine. . . . Some individual parasites, like those causing sleeping sickness, may change their coats regularly to avoid detection. Mobilizing the immune system to destroy pathogens wearing one coat is not terribly useful if parasites with different coats are continually being generated [as is the case with HIV].[21]

What a vaccine does, in other words, is stimulate the immune system to fight off this specific non-self invader when it tries to get a foothold in the body. Unfortunately, says Ewald, "the available data suggest that a person's immunological defenses are a surmountable obstacle for HIV".[22]

Still, in spite of these quite serious barriers to hope, the work to create a vaccine is still being engaged.

Why? I believe the reason is this: If HIV is indeed the etiologic agent for AIDS,[23] and if a vaccine that effectively protected against HIV were to be discovered, and if that vaccine protected a high proportion of those who were vaccinated with it, and if the vaccine were inexpensive, easily transportable, easily storable, easily administered and required only one or two doses, perhaps three at the most, then that vaccine would be an enormous benefit to humankind.[24]

Besides, there have always been skeptics and nay-sayers, people who were convinced that the improbable was really impossible. Nay-sayers criticized Wilbur and Orville Wright, vociferously characterizing their belief in the possibility of heavier-than-air flight as absurd and a foolish waste of time. They also mocked Edward Jenner and his belief that cowpox inoculation could protect people against smallpox infection. Furthermore, skeptics always seem to have plentiful evidence on their side, and numerous cases of failure to which they can point.

But sometimes the skeptics are wrong. And when they are, the believers should take credit for having had the courage to persevere with their research.

At the Tenth International Conference on AIDS in Yokohama in August 1994, Dr William Paul, head of the US Office of AIDS Research, stressed that "Despite recent setbacks, an AIDS vaccine still offers the best hope for stopping the epidemic."[25] Other investigators say in even stronger language, "the HIV vaccine research effort is of compelling public health importance."[26] While some thinkers may be concerned about the ethical propriety of expending so much money, time, and effort on vaccine development projects about which so many scientists have so many doubts, Dr Dani Bolognesi at the Duke University Medical Center explains that the "biomedical establishment cannot become passive or discouraged" by these doubts and obstacles. Instead, we need "to redouble our efforts and be prepared to maintain a long-term, solid commitment until an effective vaccine against this devastating pathogen is achieved".[27]

Perhaps precisely because a vaccine would be such a benefit, and everyone knows that it would be, HIV vaccine research is still going on. Two Seattle researchers express the feelings of many in the AIDS research community when they say that "the rapid development and testing of an HIV vaccine seems to be the highest priority research in the field of HIV."[28]

Furthermore, despite all the difficulties and research obstacles (some few of which have been detailed above), there still have been enough successes in the research to produce a small number of candidate vaccines for trials with human subjects. Some of these candidate vaccines have actually gone to phase I, and some to phase II, human trials. All of these have been of the subunit variety.

NOTES

1. C. Siebert. ""Smallpox is Dead, Long Live Smallpox." *The New York Times Magazine* 21 August 1994. section 6, 31–55, p 36.
2. S. L. Plotkin and S. A. Plotkin. "A Short History of Vaccination." *Vaccines.* Eds. S. A. Plotkin and E. A. Mortimer, second ed. (Philadelphia, PA: W.B. Saunders Co, 1994) 1–11, p 1.
3. Thucydides. *The History of the Peloponnesian War.* Vol. 6 of *Great Books of the Western World.* Trans. Crawley, Richard, and Feetham, R. 6 of 54, (Chicago: Encyclopedia Britannica, 1952) 267, p 400.
4. Quoted in S. A. Plotkin MD and E. A. Mortimer Jr, MD, eds. *Vaccines,* second ed. (Philadelphia: W.B. Saunders Company, 1994) 996+xix, p xiii.
5. However: "For more than 70 years after Edward Jenner's discovery, the world was still unaware of the existence of germs or microorganisms. It was therefore quite a leap for some to accept that they could protect themselves against one dreaded disease by being injected with another that infects cows." C. Siebert. ""Smallpox is Dead, Long Live Smallpox." *The New York Times Magazine* 21 August 1994, section 6, 31–55, p 36.
6. "Vaccinate" is from the Latin "vacca" for "cow," because the first successfully tested vaccine was against the smallpox virus, and the vaccinating pathogen that was introduced into the body was the cowpox virus. To be more specific, what was introduced, by Dr Edward Jenner, was actually pus from the sores on the wrist of a milkmaid infected with cowpox. Vaccinees did get moderately sick from cowpox, but when they healed from that, they were then protected from contracting smallpox.

   The procedure called "variolation" – variola was the medical name for smallpox – involved inoculating the individual with the actual smallpox virus.

   Vaccination is also sometimes called "inoculation," from the Latin "oculum," for eye. I thought it was named after an "oculum" because the small scar left on a person's arm – I still have such a scar – is round and looks a bit like an eye. But I discover that Klein's *Comprehensive Etymological Dictionary of the English Language,* Elsevier,

Amsterdam, 1971, says that the word derives from the past participle of "inoculare, to engraft an eye or bud from one tree into another, to implant, to furnish with eyes. From oculus, eye, bud." An inoculation, then, implants or grafts one organism into another.

The word "immune" is from the Latin immunis, "exempt from public service, free from taxes; exempt, free," formed from in- "not," and -munis, from the stem of munia (pl), "duties, services," which is related to the Latin com-munis, common." All this from Klein's, p 368.

For further discussion of smallpox vaccination, see my manuscript *Jenner on Trial: An Ethical Examination of Vaccine Research in the Age of smallpox and the Age of AIDS.*

7. At least, that is how preventive vaccines work, and that is the sort of vaccine with which this book is concerned. There are also "therapeutic vaccines" which are designed to stimulate the immune system of someone already infected with a disease. There are no such vaccines for HIV infection yet, however. There is also, at least conceptually, the possibility of a "pre-natal vaccine," i.e., a vaccine that would be designed to protect the unborn fetus from becoming infected with its mother's HIV disease. Fetuses may become infected by their mothers either in utero, or during parturition, or post partum, via breast milk. The likelihood of an HIV infected mother passing the infection to her child in one of these three ways seems to be around 20–40%. Research on pre-natal vaccines would present another assortment of ethical issues which will not be dealt with in this book.
8. "Many of the infected cells in semen and blood [i.e., cell-associated transmission] may not be destroyed because their membranes do not contain any of the viral fragments that the destroying cells use to recognize infected cells." P. Ewald. *The Evolution of Infectious Disease* (Oxford University Press, 1994), p 176.

   Also: "In these forms the virus is protected from the effects of the host's immune system and, like variability, this is a property which helps the virus to evade the immune response of the host. In this case the virus would be largely 'invisible' to the host's immune system." B. D. Schoub. *AIDS & HIV in Perspective* (New York, NY: Cambridge University Press, 1994) 268+xx, p 189.
9. P. Ewald. *The Evolution of Infectious Disease* (Oxford University Press, 1994), p 176. Also "Viral propagation in cell culture is 100- to 1000-fold greater when transmission occurs through cell fusion than through infection by free virus." p 126.
10. B. D. Schoub. *AIDS & HIV in Perspective* (New York, NY: Cambridge University Press, 1994) 268+xx, p 189.
11. J. Mann, D. Tarantola and T. Netter, eds. *AIDS in the World* (Cambridge, MA: Harvard University Press, 1992) 1037+xvi, p 33.
12. SIV is very closely related to HIV, however, so these successes are considered significant. One researcher, in fact, in trying to emphasize the similarities between SIV and HIV says "When you get down to it, there's no such thing as SIV and HIV.... It's the same virus.... We've seriously talked about calling them all PIV – Primate Immunodeficiency

Viruses, because that's what they are." D. Blum. *The Monkey Wars* (New York, NY: Oxford University Press, 1994) 306+xii, p 215.

Still, this scientist's statement notwithstanding, the international commission on virus nomenclature chose to give these two classes of virus two different names, and presumably not only because the viruses are found in two different primate species. There are other viruses that are found both in simians and humans – Ebola Marburg, Ebola Zaire, and other such filo viruses – that are not given two different names simply because they appear in two different species. There must be notable structural differences between HIV and SIV that resulted in the commission assigning two different names to the two different viruses.

13. D. Blum. *The Monkey Wars* (New York, NY: Oxford University Press, 1994) 306+xii, p 210. See also D. Hodel and AIDS Action Foundation Working Group. *HIV Preventive Vaccines: Social, Ethical, and Political Considerations* (AIDS Action Foundation, Office of AIDS Research, National Institutes of Health, 1994), p 5.
14. Unless you are using some other criterion for vaccine effectiveness besides prevention of disease.
15. D. Blum. *The Monkey Wars* (New York, NY: Oxford University Press, 1994) 306+xii, p 212.
16. B. D. Schoub. *AIDS & HIV in Perspective* (New York, NY: Cambridge University Press, 1994) 268+xx, pp 192–94.
17. D. Blum. *The Monkey Wars* (New York, NY: Oxford University Press, 1994) 306+xii , p 213.
18. *Ibid.*, p 211.
19. R. J. Levine. *Ethics and Regulation of Clinical Research*, second ed. (New Haven, CT: Yale University Press, 1986, 1988) 452+xx, p 42.

    And as Schoub says, we "need to be very cautious in not extrapolating too closely from animal model studies." B. D. Schoub. *AIDS & HIV in Perspective* (New York, NY: Cambridge University Press, 1994) 268+xx, p. 196.
20. S. Barnet, et al., "An AIDS-like Condition Induced in Baboons by HIV-2," *Science*, 266, No 5185, October 28 (1994) 642.
21. P. Ewald. *The Evolution of Infectious Disease* (Oxford University Press, 1994), p 207.
22. *Ibid.*, p 175.
23. cf Chapter 5 above.
24. Notice all the "ifs" in this paragraph; most of them are neither assured nor even very likely.
25. *The Seattle Times*, 9 August 1994, p A3.
26. D. F. Hoth, et al., "HIV Vaccine Development: A Progress Report," *Annals of Internal Medicine*, 8, 7.15 October (1994) 603–11, p 609.
27. Cotton, "International Disunity on HIV Vaccine Efficacy Trials", *JAMA*, 272, 14.12 October (1994) 1990–91, p 1091.
28. M. J. McElrath and L. Corey. "Current Status of Vaccines for HIV." *Pediatric AIDS: The challenge of HIV infection in infants, children and adolescents.* Eds. P. H. Pizzo and C. M. Wilfert (Baltimore, MD: Williams and Wilkins, 1994) 869–887, p 884.

8 Human Trials

If a candidate vaccine has shown some potential, in laboratory studies, to stimulate a successful immune response against HIV, and if it has shown the same potential in animal studies, then the vaccine may be approved for studies using human subjects.

The internationally accepted standard for vaccine research involving human subjects typically requires that human trials be done in three phases:

Phase I studies usually involve only a few human subjects, perhaps 50–80, all of whom are healthy subjects. In HIV vaccine studies, subjects in phase I trials will also probably have no known risk factors or behaviors.[1] The primary purpose of these studies is to determine safety of the vaccine in a human population. This phase may also include studies of other biological effects, perhaps including immunogenicity. These studies may last perhaps a year. If this phase is successful, candidate vaccines will go on to phase II trials.

Phase II trials continue to study safety, but the additional foci of this phase are also dosage and immunogenicity, i.e., proper dosage levels, and effectiveness in stimulating some kind of immune response. Phase II studies usually involve several hundred volunteers, perhaps up to 1000 or more (some of whom may be slightly at risk for infection),[2] and may last approximately two years. If a candidate vaccine shows promise in phase II trials as well, it may then go on to be tested in phase III trials.

Phase III trials, sometimes called efficacy trials, are "intended for a more complete assessment of safety and effectiveness in the prevention of disease, involving a larger number of volunteers in a multicentre adequately controlled study".[3] In order to be statistically meaningful, this phase will likely involve several thousand subjects, perhaps even tens of thousands, and will probably last for a minimum of three years.

In the case of HIV candidate vaccines, however, phase III trials will probably last at least four years and possibly much longer. The length of phase III trials will depend to some extent on what are considered to be the "criteria of success" for the candidate vaccine. If one criterion of effectiveness for a successful vaccine is the prevention of disease (which it doubtless will be), then phase III trials could conceivably last 15 to 20 years or more. After all, it is commonly said that the average length of time from first infection with HIV to development of formally defined AIDS is approximately 10 years. If there is any -truth to that assertion, then researchers would not know whether disease had been prevented until the 10 years had passed (plus, at a minimum, an additional two to four years) and the vaccinated subjects had not become sick.[4] (For a fuller discussion of "criteria of effectiveness" in vaccine trials, see Chapter 9.)

This commonly seen 10 year estimate, however, is only a very rough "average," in the loosest sense of the term. "A person has about a 50/50 chance of developing AIDS within 10 years after becoming infected, but the timing of this progression varies greatly from person to person."[5] That is almost an understatement. The actual time from infection to development of disease can vary from individual to individual by a factor of 12 or more. One person may become infected with HIV and develop AIDS within months while others are known to have been HIV positive for more than 13 years without progression to disease (the so-called long-term non-progressors). What accounts for such a wide disparity of experience? What cofactors might be involved in those who progress to disease rapidly? As one might imagine, this question is the subject of intense study among AIDS researchers. Some cofactors that have been considered potentially significant are route of infection, strains of the virus which are more or less virulent, cell-free vs cell-associated mode of infection, general state of the infected individual's health, presence of other causes of immunosuppression (e.g., malnutrition, infection with multiple pathogens, drug-related immunosuppression, etc.), presence of mycobacteria, quality of nutrition, exercise, and so on.

In addition, though I have not seen studies which address this question, it seems likely that the average length of time from infection to disease may well vary from country to country. If it is the case (as it seems to be) that the average length of time from infection to disease varies with the subtype and strain of HIV that has infected a person, and if the subtypes and strains of HIV vary from country to country, then it would seem likely that the average length of time from infection to disease would also vary from country to country.

If that is so, then good research protocol would require that prior epidemiological studies be conducted in nations where vaccine trials will take place, in order to determine ahead of time what the average length of time is from infection to disease. Then – again assuming that the standard for vaccine efficacy is prevention of disease – the length of vaccine trials should be that average length of time, plus some additional period of time, say another two to five years. After that fullness of time has elapsed, researchers could then declare that this candidate vaccine at least postpones the development of disease in the vaccinees, and perhaps even prevents disease altogether.

As of late 1994 "more than 1500 volunteers have been enrolled in 18 federally sponsored trials involving 13 experimental vaccines" in the US.[6] These phase I and II trials are mostly being done in the country of origin (where the vaccine was developed), which is ethically required, as we will see below. Phase I and II trials of some candidate vaccines are already being conducted in Brazil and Thailand in order to confirm the results of the phase I and II trials being done in the US.[7] Some phase III trials may also be conducted in the vaccine's country of origin, as required by the CIOMS *Ethical Guidelines.* These *Guidelines* state that in general, and unless there are good reasons for making an exception, "Phase III vaccine trials . . . should be conducted simultaneously in the host community and the sponsoring country."[8] In the case of HIV vaccines there may well be, for reasons we will explore later, good reasons for allowing that most of the phase III vaccine trials, and even the first ones, be conducted in developing communities, particularly in those communities with a high incidence of new HIV infections.

If a candidate vaccine is found, upon completion of phase III trials, to be both safe and efficacious to a satisfactory degree, this may result in eventual licensure of the vaccine and deployment into the public health arena.

I have mentioned "prevention of disease" as one of the possible standards for what would count as an effective vaccine. This is not the only, or even the most desirable, standard, as we will see in the next chapter. But whatever the chosen standard of effectiveness turns out to be, the likely prospect of a successful HIV vaccine, fully tested and ready for world wide use, is, even under the most optimistic of circumstances, several years away.

NOTES

1. S. S. Connor. "International Legal and Ethical Aspects of Developing and Distributing an HIV Vaccine." *Ethics and Law in the Study of AIDS.* Eds. H. Fuenzalida-Puelma, A. M. L. Parada and D. S. LaVertu. (Washington, DC: Pan American Health Organization, Regional Office of the World Health Organization, 1992) 162–69, p 165.
2. D. Hodel and AIDS Action Foundation Working Group. *HIV Preventive Vaccines: Social, Ethical, and Political Considerations* (AIDS Action Foundation, Office of AIDS Research, National Institutes of Health, 1994), p 6.
3. Z. Bankowski and R. J. Levine, eds. *Ethics and Research on Human Subjects: International Guidelines (Proceedings of the XXVIth CIOMS Conference, Geneva, Switzerland, 5–7 February 1992).* (Geneva, Switzerland: Council for International Organizations of Medical Sciences (CIOMS), 1993) 228+63+x, p 51.
4. However, Dr Peter Piot tells me that this 10 year estimate of HIV latency is a bit too long. "The current accepted estimate of HIV latency is a median of 7 years, and a trial with disease as an end point can be done in less than 10 years," Personal communication, 20 December 1995.
5. P. Ewald. *The Evolution of Infectious Disease* (New York, NY: Oxford University Press, 1994) 298+x, p 163.
6. L. K. Altman MD. "After Setback, First Large AIDS Vaccine Trials Are Planned." *New York Times* 29 November 1994, B6.

   B. D. Schoub. *AIDS & HIV in Perspective* (New York, NY: Cambridge University Press, 1994) 268+xx, p 196–97. Also M. J. McElrath and L. Corey. "Current Status of Vaccines for HIV." *Pediatric AIDS: The challenge of HIV infection in infants, children and adolescents.* Eds. P. H. Pizzo and C. M. Wilfert (Baltimore, MD: Williams and Wilkins, 1994) 869–887, p 878.

Hoth, et al. say that the number was actually closer to 1600 volunteers, by August 1994. D. F. Hoth, et al., "HIV Vaccine Development: A Progress Report," *Annals of Internal Medicine*, 8, 7.15 October (1994) 603–11, p. 609.

For a list of the twelve candidate vaccines already under study in early 1992, cf J. Mann, D. Tarantola and T. Netter, eds. *AIDS in the World* (Cambridge, MA: Harvard University Press, 1992) 1037+xvi, p 248.

7. Cotton, "International Disunity on HIV Vaccine Efficacy Trials," *JAMA*, 272, 14.12 October (1994) 1090–91, p 1091.
8. CIOMS Ethical Guidelines require that phase III trials be conducted in the country of origin before, or at the same time as, they are conducted in developing nations. Z. Bankowski and R. J. Levine, eds. *Ethics and Research on Human Subjects: International Guidelines (Proceedings of the XXVIth CIOMS Conference, Geneva, Switzerland, 5–7 February 1992).* (Geneva, Switzerland: Council for International Organizations of Medical Sciences (CIOMS), 1993) 228+63+x. Commentary on Guideline 8, p 27.

It would seem questionable, however, if phase III vaccine testing in the industrialized West were to be "delayed until the correlates of protection (see Chapter 9, below) – or clear markers of protection – are understood." Yet this possibility is considered in P. Cotton, "International Disunity on Vaccine Efficacy Trials", *JAMA*, 272, Number 14, 12 October (1994) 1090.

9 Criteria of Effectiveness

9.1 WHAT DOES "VACCINE SUCCESS" MEAN?

What should be considered the standard or criterion of a successful preventive HIV vaccine? Or to phrase the question a bit differently, what exactly is it that we want a vaccine to accomplish? The simple answer is that what we want from a vaccine is for it to protect us from contracting a certain disease. But how exactly do we want it to protect us from that disease, and how will we determine whether it has accomplished that? What criteria will we use to determine whether we have a successful vaccine or not? Four possible criteria have been considered:

1 The emergence of certain measurable markers in the immune system, such as the emergence of certain kinds of antibodies or certain kinds of T-cells,[1] for example, could be treated as an indication that the vaccine is a success. This result – usually termed immunogenicity, i.e., the generation of a measurable immune response – has actually already been achieved in most of the first generation of candidate vaccines in phase I and II testing right now. This criterion of success, a rather weak one by anyone's measure, is actually part of what is being looked for in every candidate vaccine during phase II trials. If the candidate vaccine cannot demonstrate that it produces any immune response at all, then it will likely not go on to phase III trials. If, on the other hand, the candidate vaccine demonstrates that it does generate some kind of immune response in phase II trials, then it may go on to phase III trials. In phase III trials we will be looking for "efficacy," i.e., for whether the candidate vaccine is actually efficacious in doing what we want it to do. If we do at some point find a vaccine that is successful, then we can retrospectively look back and try to correlate the kinds of immune responses we saw in phase II trials with the efficacy of the vaccine discovered in phase III trials. We would then have determined what "the correlates of protection" are, and this would be an enormous step

forward in vaccine research. At that point we would then know what the immune system needs to do in order to beat this virus.

Unfortunately, as of yet, no one knows which immune system markers will be indicative of a successful vaccine. *JAMA* reports in August 1994 that "despite extraordinary research efforts aimed at understanding the immunology of HIV-1, the immune correlates of protection remain unknown."[2] And *Science* reports in September of 1994 that "no researcher has yet demonstrated which immune responses provide protection."[3] This unhappy state of affairs means that immune system markers, though they should undoubtedly be monitored and correlated with future findings of progression (or non-progression) to disease, are not yet adequate endpoints for a vaccine study.[4]

But even if the "correlates of protection" were known, we would still need to clarify exactly what it is that we want a vaccine to do, i.e., how exactly we want it to protect us.

So what is it that we want a vaccine to accomplish?

2 What we would most like a vaccine to accomplish is to "prevent infection," i.e., to prevent our even becoming infected with the agent that causes the disease. This is a very high standard, however. A vaccine which met this standard would have the following effect: it would generate such a strong response in the vaccinee's immune system that when that vaccinee is later exposed to a wild virus (assuming that a virus is the etiologic agent of the disease we are protecting against), the immune system would immediately recognize that wild virus as the invader for which it had been primed and which it should fight off. The immune system would then immediately, or almost immediately, go into action and within a short time would successfully eliminate all traces of the virus, both free virus and cell-associated virus, from the vaccinee's body. If the immune system acted immediately in such a way as to block any sort of initial infection, this would be termed "sterilizing immunity." If the immune system allowed a brief infection but then cleared it out almost immediately, this would also be termed "preventing infection." In either case, the virus would never get a foothold in the body. All traces of it would be completely eliminated. The immune system would have successfully prevented

the vaccinee from being infected with that virus. It would have protected the person from infection.[5]

We could determine whether the vaccine had been successful according to this criterion by testing for two events: a) determining whether the vaccinee had been exposed to a wild virus, and b) determining whether there are now any traces of that wild virus still remaining anywhere in the vaccinee's body.[6] If there are not any such traces, then we could say that that vaccine had met this standard and had prevented infection.

However, even if a candidate HIV vaccine did successfully meet this high standard and did prevent infection with wild virus, this first generation (at least) of vaccine trials would still need to follow their subjects for several more years (or even, possibly, for the rest of their lives) to insure that they still do not come down with AIDS.[7] No matter how obvious it may seem, it cannot be simply assumed, *a priori*, that prevention (actually, elimination) of HIV infection necessarily also prevents subsequent disease. Subjects would still need to be monitored to discover whether this form of preventing HIV infection was also successful in preventing the disease of AIDS or not.

In any case, what we would truly like a vaccine to do is to prevent infection with the virus. This is a very high standard of success, however. Some would say it is an almost impossibly high standard, and not likely to be achieved. Whether this outcome is likely or not is what remains to be determined by efficacy trials.

Suppose, however, that a vaccine is not able to meet this high standard. What, then, is the next best thing that we would like a vaccine to accomplish?

3 The next best thing we would like from a vaccine, if it cannot successfully prevent infection, is that it would at least prevent disease. This is the most historically common criterion of success in vaccines for other infectious diseases. That is to say, vaccines in use against today's common viral diseases (polio, for example) "generally work to prevent disease without preventing subclinical infection."[8] If a vaccine were to meet this more common standard of success, it would mean that the effect it had on the vaccinee was as follows: upon being vaccinated, the subject's immune system would

respond, would gear up for this viral invader, and would be primed for the fight. Then, when exposed to the wild virus, it would not actually prevent infection with the virus but instead would allow infection, yet would keep the virus "in check." That is, the immune system would allow the virus to have a foothold in the body, but would be able to successfully keep that virus from replicating, or at least from causing any clinical symptoms of disease. In this way, the vaccinee's immune system would be able to prevent the virus from ever causing any damage in the body.

This kind of successful vaccine, if it were able to keep the virus in check and able to prevent or reduce viral replication, may also have the simultaneous effect of reducing the "viral load," i.e., reducing the total amount of virus in the vaccinee's body, both free virus in the blood and other bodily fluids, and the cell-associated virus inside human cells.[9] This effect then could also result in a lesser degree of viral transmission from the vaccinee to others with whom the vaccinee might have contact. This lower degree of transmission would then be a secondary benefit of this kind of vaccine. This kind of vaccine may also have the effect of preventing the significant decline in T4 (CD4) cells that is so characteristic of HIV infection, and which seems to signal the diminishing effectiveness of an infected person's immune system.[10]

This successful outcome, i.e., allowing subclinical infection but preventing clinical disease, could be determined to have occurred by observing for four different factors: a) testing to determine whether the vaccinee had indeed been exposed to a wild virus, b) testing to determine whether the immune system is efficiently keeping viral replication in check (i.e., whether the total viral load has been reduced in the vaccinee's cells, blood and other bodily fluids), c) observing the CD4 count to see whether it remains stable over time, and d) observing the vaccinee for the remainder of his or her life to see that no immune-related disease ever develops. This would take many years, of course, as we have seen earlier, but if all four of these factors were to be observed, that would mean the vaccine had proven successful in protecting a person from disease.

A person who had been vaccinated with a vaccine of this sort and then had been exposed to HIV could then know that they would never get sick from the infection. This, of course, would be very good news for them.

We should also ask, however, (clinically and dispassionately) what public health effect the licensure and deployment of such a vaccine might have on the future course of the HIV/AIDS pandemic. One effect it would have is that the HIV+ person might then not feel so badly about being infected. They would, after all, be fully protected (*ex hypothesi*) against ever getting sick from that virus. That would be a great advantage to the individual vaccinee.

The disadvantage of this scenario, however, in terms of its effect on the pandemic, is that those vaccinees who had been exposed to HIV and who had become infected by it, would still be contagious and therefore capable of passing the virus on to others. This circumstance could have the paradoxical effect of actually worsening the epidemic by resulting in a larger number of still contagious, longer-living persons with HIV, thereby increasing the total global viral pool. That is to say, with the deployment of a vaccine of this sort, "viral spread may continue unabated, or even intensify."[11] Thus, the public health benefit of a hypothetically reduced viral load in the vaccinee may be completely offset by the large increase in the number of years that the disease-free individual would continue to be contagious and capable of transmitting the virus to others. Many traditional vaccines that allow infection but prevent disease do not have this same problem. When those other vaccines prevent disease, they also thereby prevent contagion, because in many diseases it is the disease process itself (with its attendant coughing, sneezing, open sores, etc.) that renders the individual contagious. Without the disease itself there is little or no contagion. But that is not the case with HIV infection. An HIV+ person may be entirely disease-free (in fact most HIV+ persons are disease-free for most of the years they are infected) and yet still be fully capable of infecting others. So an HIV vaccine that allowed infection but prevented disease would not be near the blessing that other vaccines are which merely prevent disease.

On the other hand, if a vaccine like this were available which did successfully prevent progression to disease (even though it did not prevent infection), then people might not mind becoming infected with HIV. If HIV infection had no negative consequences at all, then being infected with it would be virtually the same thing as not being infected with it, as long as people had been vaccinated with this (hypothetical) disease-preventing vaccine.[12]

(In addition, a preventive vaccine of this sort which had this ability to protect infected persons from disease might also work to some extent as a therapeutic vaccine. That is, in addition to the vaccine's effectiveness as a prophylactic to non-infected persons, it might also prove beneficial to persons who have already become infected. It might be able to prevent disease from developing even in those persons already infected. Important work is already being done on the possibility of therapeutic vaccines, but it will not be dealt with here. "Ethically and socially, the dilemmas posed by therapeutic vaccine development resemble more closely those [dilemmas] posed by the development of drugs and other treatments,"[13] and, important as they are, those issues are not the focus of this book.)

However, suppose a vaccine is not able to meet even this standard of success, i.e., is not able to prevent infection, and is not even able to prevent disease. What would then be the next best thing we would like a vaccine to do?

4 The next best thing we would like a vaccine to do is to prime our immune system so that it can at least fight off the virus to some extent. Even if the vaccine is not able to completely prevent disease, perhaps it will at least be able to effectively postpone disease and protect a person for a while. Or if not that, then perhaps the vaccine could at least ameliorate the disease processes so that AIDS and other HIV disease would not be nearly as gruesome as they are now.

A vaccine of this sort which postponed the onset of disease or attenuated the disease process itself would at least provide some minor degree of protection for the individual, and would at least be better than nothing (for individuals). As for the public health effect on the pandemic of a vaccine of this sort, it could increase the spread of HIV due to an increase in the years of possible contagion. One researcher suggests that a vaccine of this sort "would be a medical success, but a public health failure."[14]

(A vaccine that met this standard could also probably be used as a therapeutic vaccine.)

This criterion of success is by far the most modest criterion. It may also be the one most likely to actually be accomplished.

In any case, what we want from a vaccine is that it be able to protect us in some measure from the effects of an encounter with wild HIV.

9.2 PER CENT EFFICACY

Another equally important question that needs to be considered is: what percentage of those who are vaccinated do we want the vaccine to protect? The answer, of course, is that ideally we would like it to protect 100 per cent of those vaccinated. No vaccine for any disease, however, meets this high standard. Most licensed vaccines range from 80 per cent to 95 per cent efficacy,[15] and we consider a rate this high to be quite good.[16] Indeed, a rate of effectiveness this high is eminently protective both of the individual who is vaccinated, and of the human "herd" in which the individual lives and moves and has his or her being. Because the vaccine protects 80 per cent to 95 per cent of the individuals in the herd, it also therefore dramatically reduces the disease pool, and therefore decreases the amount of the disease in the population as a whole. Therefore it improves the chances of even unvaccinated persons for being protected against infection. So a vaccine that is 80 to 95 per cent effective is actually extremely beneficial both to the individual and to the herd. An HIV vaccine that was 80 per cent to 95 per cent effective would go a very long ways toward controlling this epidemic.

However, the likelihood of finding an HIV vaccine that is anywhere near that effective is not very high. Most researchers are hoping for a vaccine that would be 50 per cent to 60 per cent effective. (Some policy makers may even find it acceptable to license and deploy an HIV vaccine that is only 30 per cent effective.) They seem to feel that a vaccine of even that limited degree of effectiveness would provide at least some modest level of protection for individuals and for society.

> Scientists and policy-makers have realized that an effective but less than "ideal" vaccine (for example, one that is effective in preventing HIV (AIDS) in 50 to 60% of vaccinated persons instead of the 80 to 95% efficacy achieved for most licensed vaccines) could still have dramatic public health benefits.[17]

I regularly see these 50 to 60 per cent efficacy estimates for potential HIV vaccines, followed, as in the above statement, by the claim that even though this is not as high as we would like an HIV vaccine's efficacy to be, at least it would still provide *some* measure of benefit to individuals and to the public health.[18] It will at least be better, according to these claims, to have a low efficacy vaccine than to have no vaccine at all.

I have seen this statement often enough that I have begun to wonder whether it is actually true that a moderately effective HIV vaccine would provide a moderately effective benefit. Might there not be at least a possibility that a moderately effective vaccine would perhaps not make any difference at all in the spread of HIV, and perhaps could even make the pandemic worse? As it turns out, this is indeed a real possibility.

9.3 COULD A VACCINE WORSEN THE EPIDEMIC?

To illustrate this possibility, consider the following brief thought-experiment:

Imagine that an HIV vaccine of very low efficacy, say 10 to 15 per cent efficacy, were to be licensed and deployed in the population. Is it not at least a conceivable consequence that

1 not very many people would choose to be vaccinated with a product that offers so little protection (and therefore it would do those unvaccinated persons no good at all); and, more importantly,
2 that those who did get vaccinated might now feel a bit safer because they had "been vaccinated." And if they did feel safer, might they not also tend to be a bit less careful about their risky behaviors, thereby putting

> themselves and others at even more risk than if they had not been vaccinated at all?

> It is also possible that if risk behavior increased as a consequence of a mass vaccination campaign, then . . .mass vaccination may have the perverse outcome of increasing the severity of the epidemic[19]

Whether such a paradoxical increase in the severity of the epidemic would actually result from the deployment of a moderately effective licensed HIV vaccine would depend on three separate factors: a) the degree of increase in risk behaviors over what those risk behaviors would have been without the introduction of the vaccine, b) the per cent efficacy of the vaccine used, and c) the "coverage" of the vaccine, i.e., the percentage of people who actually get vaccinated. In the *Science* article referred to just above, Blower and McLean report a study which shows, not surprisingly, that the lower the efficacy level of a vaccine, the fewer people are likely to choose to be vaccinated. Their study then concludes that

> a mass vaccination campaign could *increase the severity of the epidemic* if it was only possible to achieve 50% coverage levels for a 60% effective vaccine and the level of the risk behavior increased by a factor of 1.4.[20]

These estimates do not seem out of line: 50 per cent coverage levels might even be a little bit optimistic; 60 per cent is certainly within the range of vaccine efficacy that researchers seem to be expecting, and an estimated 1.4 increase in risk behaviors (not anywhere near 2.0, or doubling) also seems relatively conservative. And yet that scenario would, if Blower's and McLean's modeling is correct,[21] have the effect of worsening the pandemic, despite the presence of a moderately successful vaccine.

This paradoxical worsening of an epidemic despite the presence of a moderately successful vaccine (if such a thing were to happen) would not be the first time in history that an inoculation program had worsened an epidemic. In 18th century England, well before Edward Jenner's experiments which tested whether cowpox inoculation could prevent smallpox, the practice of variolation had become popular.

Variolation was the practice of inoculating people with actual smallpox "virus"[22] in hopes that they would contract only a very mild case of the disease, and then that they would thereafter be immune from later ever contracting a more serious case of smallpox disease.[23] This practice was moderately successful at immunizing individuals against contracting subsequent smallpox disease, but it probably also had the paradoxical public health effect of actually worsening smallpox epidemics by increasing the number of temporarily contagious people.[24] (Edward Jenner's discovery, of course, was that inoculation with another disease toxin which was much less pathogenic – the cowpox "virus" – could also immunize people against infection with smallpox. Whether there could be any analogs here for AIDS vaccine research is as yet completely unknown.)

This potential worsening of the AIDS pandemic as a result of having and deploying an AIDS vaccine is, I believe, worth considering. It may imply that what we really need is an HIV vaccine that is much more than 60 per cent effective in its protection of vaccinees. Or, if it does not imply that, it may simply be a stark reminder that any successful solution to the AIDS pandemic will need to include a continued and probably even intensified insistence on large scale reduction in risk behaviors. A vaccine alone, particularly one that is only 60 per cent or so effective, will probably not by itself help slow the pandemic.[25]

These questions about which standards of effectiveness to use are crucial questions. Which of the three main criteria of effectiveness should we be aiming for: prevention of infection, prevention of disease, or attenuation/postponement of disease? The highest criterion, of course. But which of these criteria should we count as acceptable if we are not able to find a vaccine that meets the highest standard? And what percentage of effectiveness should we be aiming for in HIV vaccines? 100 per cent effectiveness, of course, but if we cannot achieve that, then what percentage of effectiveness should we deem acceptable?

9.4 STANDARDS FOR VACCINE LICENSURE

Even though these questions are of crucial importance, there are as yet no agreed upon answers to them. Dr Wayne Koff recommends in a recent article in *Science*,[26] that an international regulatory commission should be established immediately to arrive (by consensus) at some answers to these questions.

> Guidance from regulatory authorities on efficacy expectations will have a critical impact on the design of the field trial itself, particularly on sample sizes (the numbers of subjects to be immunized) necessary to determine vaccine efficacy. Is a target of 50 to 60% [efficacy] realistic for licensure [of a vaccine]? Is protection against 50 to 60% of the major circulating subtypes of HIV sufficient for licensure? Is protection for 1 year, with the requirement for an annual booster immunization sufficient for licensure? . . . An international regulatory consensus on the expected levels of vaccine efficacy would accelerate the timetable for licensing a globally effective AIDS vaccine.[27]

I fully concur with Dr Koff's call for an international regulatory commission to make recommendations on standards for vaccine licensure. Without such a set of standards, vaccine developers cannot even be sure what they should be aiming for, and cannot know what results licensing agencies are likely to find acceptable.

I also concur with Dr Koff that it should be done now, rather than some years from now. The progress of science is slow, and by nature must be slow. The growth and movement of governmental agencies, especially inter-governmental agencies, is also slow, but it is not necessarily and by nature slow. In times of urgent need governments can and do move quickly. This is one time they should.

9.5 URGENCY: A DOUBLE-EDGED SWORD

There is, after all, a real urgency. In Northern Thailand, for example, where $60 million has already been spent on

AIDS prevention, and the annual incidence of new infections is still accelerating, there is a sense of desperation. "We *need* a vaccine," the Thai government has told the World Health Organization.[28]

This sense of urgency is further underscored by a strong consensus among the world's leading vaccinologists. A survey of 100 leading vaccinologists concluded that a vaccine against HIV was urgently needed soon. In the September 2, 1994 issue of *Science*, editors reported on their survey of "an international sample of more than 100 of [vaccinology's] leading researchers, public health officials, and manufacturers. All told, 67 people from 18 countries on six continents responded [to this survey]." Besides the consensus among respondents that the field of vaccinology lacked both strong leadership and adequate funding, there was also a strong consensus that a vaccine for HIV was the highest vaccine priority in the world, and that it was urgently needed soon.

> The survey . . . asked respondents to list, in order of priority, the most urgently needed new vaccines, listing the developing and developed countries separately. [A] strong consensus put an AIDS vaccine at the top of the list for both developing and developed countries.[29]

There is little doubt that an HIV vaccine that protected against infection, or even one that protected only against the development of AIDS, could be an important boost in the struggle to contain this pandemic. In many developing nations, the epidemic's numbers are growing very rapidly, even accelerating, as time passes. If there are not developed soon effective preventive measures which are much more successful than those used so far, the long term global effects could be dramatic.

This sense of urgency, however, is a double-edged sword. It is both a blessing and a danger. As a blessing, it strongly motivates researchers to put their best efforts into the achievement of a goal that sometimes looks impossible. Petriciani, Koff and Ada, for example, argue passionately for pressing on with efficacy trials:

> Proceeding . . . with clinical efficacy trials should not be considered adventurism, but rather a pragmatic approach

to gain the most meaningful type of information as soon as possible. It is the way to progress in the best tradition of past vaccine efforts such as those against smallpox, rabies, and polio. The world is a healthier place today because individuals dedicated to attacking those diseases took the initiative to move ahead and learn from clinical studies.

A recent editorial in the *Lancet* described the problem of tuberculosis in HIV-infected persons in Africa as one of the greatest public health disasters since the bubonic plague. In discussing what might be done to deal with the situation, the point was made that the time for elegant studies and perfection is past, and that sights must be set on practical targets – not idealized goals. We should do no less in the HIV vaccine field.[30]

As a danger, however, the urgency brings with it a serious risk: that researchers may want to cut corners, may become over-hasty in their studies, and may even be willing to overlook certain ethical guidelines here or there if those guidelines appear less important than the rapid development of a workable vaccine. Even at a recent conference on human rights which I attended (at which some of the ideas in this book were presented) some of the participants (all of whom were intelligent and caring academics) seemed surprisingly willing to abrogate some of the ethical principles that guide human subjects research. If even some of these well-educated humanists, committed as they are to the goals of human rights and the compassionate treatment of all human beings, might be willing to allow the cutting of ethical corners, how might some others feel who are working on the front lines of the pandemic and who are daily faced with this sense of high urgency?

This is the concern of those who hold the Antithesis position. It is absolutely imperative, in their minds, that any persons who volunteer to participate as subjects in vaccine trials be fully informed, and that their rights be fully protected, in full accord with all internationally accepted ethical standards for human subjects research.

What are these ethical standards for human subjects research, where can we find them, and how do they apply to HIV vaccine trials? It is to these questions that we will now turn our attention.

NOTES

1. As, for example, cytotoxic T-lymphocytes, or CTL cells, which seem to be significant in the control of HIV infection, particularly with cell-associated virus. These CTL cells, however, seem to be much more difficult to induce, particularly with subunit vaccines. W. N. Rida and D. N. Lawrence, "Some Statistical Issues in HIV Vaccine Trials," *Statistics in Medicine,* 13 (1994) 2155–77, pp 2159, 2169.
2. J. R. Mascola MD, J. G. McNeil MD, MPH and D. S. Burke MD, "AIDS Vaccines: Are We Ready for Human Efficacy Trials?," *Journal of the American Medical Association,* 272, 6, August 10 (1994) 488–89, p 489.

   What are some of the contenders for what the correlates of immunity might be? Some think the answer lies in the production of antibodies, others think the answer lies in the production of cytotoxic T-lymphocytes (CTLs), still others think the answer lies in mucosal immunity

   > in which the virus is attacked when it passes the mucus membranes that line the entrances to the body. And some think any vaccine must produce all three. 'The whole (scientific) community seems to be fragmented right now as to what they think a vaccine is supposed to be,' says Dani Bolognesi, a highly regarded AIDS vaccine expert at Duke University who serves on the AIDS research council. 'None of us know what it is going to take to do this.' S. Stolberg. "Promise, Disappointment Mark AIDS Vaccine Quest." *Los Angeles Times* 9 August 1994, A1.

3. J. Cohen, "Bumps on the Vaccine Road," *Science,* 265, 2 September (1994) 1371–73, p 1373. This weekly journal of the American Association for the Advancement of Science devoted this number of the journal to a variety of articles and studies on current issues in vaccinology.
4. Those who do research with BCG vaccine (for tuberculosis) are faced with the same problem. "The exact immunological mechanisms that characterize human resistance and reaction to *M. tuberculosis* remain largely undetermined." J. R. Starke and K. K. Connelly. "Bacille Calmette-Guérin Vaccine." *Vaccines,* eds S. A. Plotkin MD and E. A. Mortimer Jr, MD, second ed. (Philadelphia: W. B. Saunders Company, 1994) 439–73, p 442.
5. This result seems to have been successfully achieved in SIV vaccines in some monkeys, however, when challenged intrarectally with low doses of live SIV. When challenged vaginally with live SIV, however, the results were not nearly as promising. The reasons for the difference were not clear. Furthermore, this study involved only 8 monkeys, and this is far too few animals to draw any meaningful conclusions. M. B. Gardner and S.-L. Hu, "SIV vaccines, 1991 – a year in review," *AIDS,* 5 (supplement 2) (1991) S115–S127, p S121.
6. There may be some difficulties involved in assessing the presence and absence of HIV in a person, because "virus may be cleared from

the peripheral circulation, but remain in lymph nodes and other tissues, making it difficult to judge if an infection has truly been eliminated." W. N. Rida and D. N. Lawrence, "Some Statistical Issues in HIV Vaccine Trials," *Statistics in Medicine,* 13 (1994) 2155–77, p 2170.

7. D. F. Hoth, et al., "HIV Vaccine Development: A Progress Report," *Annals of Internal Medicine,* 8, 7.15 October (1994) 603–11, p 608.
8. P. Stehr-green. personal communication about vaccines. 4 January 1995. Dr Stehr-green is an epidemiologist with the Washington State Department of Public Health in Olympia, WA.

   Also, "This infection-permissive type of immunization is considered the predominant mode of action of most viral vaccines." M. B. Gardner and S.-L. Hu, "SIV vaccines, 1991 – a year in review," *AIDS,* 5 (supplement 2) (1991) S115–S127, p S123.

   "Traditionally, most vaccines have prevented disease rather than infection." W. N. Rida and D. N. Lawrence, "Some Statistical Issues in HIV Vaccine Trials," *Statistics in Medicine,* 13 (1994) 2155–77, p 2160.

   "Most vaccines prevent disease, not infection." B. F. Haynes, "Scientific and Social Issues of Human Immunodeficiency Virus Vaccine Development," *Science,* 260.28 May (1993) 1279–86, p 1279.

   Also, "BCG vaccination [for tuberculosis] does not prevent infection with M. tuberculosis, but helps the host to retard the growth of organisms at the primary site of infection and prevent massive lymphohematogenous dissemination."J. R. Starke and K. K. Connelly. "Bacille Calmette-Guérin Vaccine." *Vaccines,* eds S. A. Plotkin MD and E. A. Mortimer Jr, MD, second ed. (Philadelphia: W.B. Saunders Company, 1994) 439–73, p 453.
9. Rida and Lawrence report that animal studies of some HIV candidate vaccines have shown a reduction in viral load in some vaccinated monkeys of up to 80 or 90%. W. N. Rida and D. N. Lawrence, "Some Statistical Issues in HIV Vaccine Trials," *Statistics in Medicine,* 13 (1994) 2155–77, p 2158.
10. D. F. Hoth, et al., "HIV Vaccine Development: A Progress Report," *Annals of Internal Medicine,* 8, 7.15 October (1994) 603–11, p 608.
11. J. Mann, D. Tarantola and T. Netter, eds. *AIDS in the World* (Cambridge, MA: Harvard University Press, 1992) 1037+xvi, pp 255–56.
12. One researcher speculates that vaccine trials in the US will probably be designed with prevention of infection as the primary objective. However, "in developing countries, where HIV incidence rates may be higher and the median incubation period for disease may be shorter, it may be feasible to study a candidate vaccine's ability to prevent or delay disease." W. N. Rida and D. N. Lawrence, "Some Statistical Issues in HIV Vaccine Trials," *Statistics in Medicine,* 13 (1994) 2155–77, p 2160.
13. D. Hodel and AIDS Action Foundation Working Group. *HIV Preventive Vaccines: Social, Ethical, and Political Considerations* (AIDS Action Foundation, Office of AIDS Research, National Institutes of Health, 1994), preface.

14. W. N. Rida and D. N. Lawrence, "Some Statistical Issues in HIV Vaccine Trials," *Statistics in Medicine,* 13 (1994) 2155–77, p 2160.
15. W. C. Koff, "The Next Steps Toward a Global AIDS Vaccine," *Science,* 266.25 November (1994) 1335–37, p 1336.
16. Moore, John, and Roy Anderson. "The WHO and why of HIV vaccine trials." *Nature* 372.24 November (1994): 313–14, p 313.
17. Koff, Wayne C. "The Next Steps Toward a Global AIDS Vaccine." *Science* 266.25 November 1994 (1994): 1335–37, 1336.
18. One respected source says, for example: ". . . even a vaccine with a relatively low level of efficacy might save large numbers of lives." in "HIV vaccines get the green light for Third World trials." *Nature* 371.20 October (1994): 644.
19. Blower, S. M., and A. R. McLean. "Prophylactic Vaccines, Risk Behavior Change, and the Probability of Eradicating HIV in San Francisco." *Science* 265.2 September (1994): 1451–1454, 1453.
20. *Ibid.* Emphasis mine.
21. I have been told by reliable sources that Blower's and McLean's mathematical modeling is not entirely satisfactory, however, so their estimates may be inaccurate. The issue, however, still seems worth considering when it comes time for public health officials to make decisions about deploying a vaccine.
22. The term "virus" was used at that time with its original Latin meaning: a poison or toxin; not with today's meaning: a tiny, quasi-living particle of genetic material with a protein coat.
23. See my *Jenner on Trial: An Ethical Examination of Vaccine Research in the Age of Smallpox and the Age of AIDS.*
24. A. J. H. Rains MS, FRCS. *Edward Jenner and Vaccination. Pioneers of Science and Discovery* (East Sussex: Wayland Publishers, 1974, 1980) 96, pp 54, 57.
25. WHO recently announced that it has been generously granted full rights to a malaria vaccine (by Dr Manuel Patarroyo, the developer of the vaccine) which is only approximately 30 per cent effective, and which the WHO will continue to study for possible deployment in Africa. However, the deployment of a 30 per cent effective malaria vaccine in a high incidence area (e.g., southern Tanzania, where persons can be subjected to 20–25 infectious mosquito bites every night) is quite a different issue than deploying a 30 per cent effective HIV vaccine, for two reasons: a) the 30 per cent effective malaria vaccine would probably be given to almost the entire population, either by mandate or by choice. And b) whereas some persons at risk for HIV infection might increase their risk behaviors due to feeling safer after being vaccinated, persons in malaria infested areas will probably not be increasing their exposure to malaria-carrying mosquitoes after they have been vaccinated. For these reasons, it might make good sense to deploy a 30 per cent effective malaria vaccine, but might not make sense to deploy a 30 per cent (or even 50 or 60 per cent) effective HIV vaccine. See WHO, *Malaria vaccine reduces disease in African children* (World Health Organization, 28 October 1994).

26. Koff, Wayne C. "The Next Steps Toward a Global AIDS Vaccine," *Science* 266.25 November (1994): 1335–37.
27. *Ibid.* p 1336.
28. P. Piot. *Lecture on Global Issues for HIV Prevention and Control.* Harborview Medical Center: University of Washington, July 13, 1994. Also: Piot says there is an "urgent need and pressure from the most affected countries to move ahead and accelerate vaccine development." Cotton, "International Disunity on HIV Vaccine Efficacy Trials," *JAMA*, 272, 14.12 October (1994) 1090–91, p 1091.
29. J. Cohen, "Bumps on the Vaccine Road," *Science*, 265.2 September (1994) 1371–73, p 1371.
30. J. C. Petricciani, W. C. Koff and G. L. Ada, "Efficacy Trials for HIV/AIDS Vaccines," *AIDS Research and Human Retroviruses*, 8, 8 (1992) 1527–29, p 1529.

10 Ethical Principles

By international agreement, all medical research which involves human beings[1] is subject to at least three overarching ethical principles:

1 The principle of *beneficence* requires that researchers, in addition to refraining from doing deliberate harm (nonmaleficence), must make every reasonable effort to maximize benefits and goods, and to minimize harms and burdens.

   This principle gives rise to norms requiring that the risks of research be reasonable in the light of the expected benefits, that the research design be sound, and that the investigators be competent both to conduct the research and to safeguard the welfare of the research subjects.[2]

2 The principle of *autonomy* derives from the principle of *respect for persons* and requires that "those who are capable of deliberation about their personal choices should be treated with respect for their capacity for self-determination."[3] This principle also requires that the rights of persons not entirely capable of self-determination be fully protected, and that vulnerable persons be made secure from harm or abuse.

3 The principle of *justice* requires that every person be given what is rightly due to them, and that the potential benefits and burdens of medical research be fairly distributed. Here too, "special provisions must be made for the protection of the rights and welfare of vulnerable persons."[4]

The importance of articulating these principles became glaringly evident during the Nuremberg Trials in Germany following World War II. The world then saw what grotesque and tragic violations of the rights of human beings could be perpetrated, even by physicians, in the name of medical science. Out of that tragic awareness came the first clearly articulated set of ethical standards for human subjects research. It was completed in 1947, and has become known as *The Nuremberg Code.* This code acknowledges that research involving human subjects is necessary, useful and good, but insists that such research is acceptable only if certain ethical principles are scrupulously adhered to.

Because the human subjects in the Nazi medical experiments had come from among prisoners in the concentration camps, and because their personal autonomy had been so cruelly violated, the principle of autonomy is the ethical axiom that is given the strongest emphasis in *The Nuremberg Code.* The first and central ethical demand in the code is that "the voluntary consent of the human subject is absolutely essential." This is the first clear statement of the principle of informed consent. We will be returning to a fuller discussion of this principle later, but for now one point needs to be emphasized: the principle of informed consent requires that each research volunteer be fully informed about the experiment in which they will be participating. Each prospective subject must be told

> the nature, duration, and purpose of the experiment; the method and means by which it is to be conducted; all inconveniences and hazards reasonably to be expected; and the effects upon his health or person which may possibly come from his participation in the experiment.[5]

In addition to being properly informed, prospective volunteers must also be able to choose freely, without any elements of deceit or coercion, whether they will participate in the research, and they must furthermore be of age, and "competent" to so decide. More on those issues later. For now, we will focus on what "inconveniences and hazards reasonably to be expected" might result from a volunteer's participation in HIV vaccine research. Some of them are not minor.

NOTES

1. Research involving animals is also subject to ethical principles, though this book does not examine those. Besides the writings of philosopher Peter Singer and others on the subject of animal rights, the

Council for International Organizations of Medical Sciences (CIOMS), based in Geneva, Switzerland, spent three years studying, consulting, writing, and then publishing a set of ethical guidelines for research involving animals. cf. Z. Bankowski, ed. *International Guiding Principles for Biomedical Research Involving Animals* (Geneva, Switzerland: Council for International Organizations of Medical Sciences (CIOMS), 1985) 28. *See also* a new book on the subject just published in late 1994: D. Blum. *The Monkey Wars* (New York, NY: Oxford University Press, 1994) 306+xii.

2. Z. Bankowski, ed. *International Ethical Guidelines for Biomedical Research Involving Human Subjects* (Geneva, Switzerland: Council for International Organizations of Medical Sciences (CIOMS), 1993) 63, p 10.
3. *Ibid.*
4. *Ibid.* p 11.
5. *Nuremberg Code,* section 1. Cf Appendix I.

11 Real Risks

A preliminary disquisition on The Other

In considering the risks detailed in the following sections, those who hold the Antithesis position would wish readers and researchers to keep in mind the wise little proverb: "The burdens that appear easiest to bear are those that are borne by others." This is particularly important to keep in mind because virtually all volunteers in phase III HIV vaccine trials will be persons from groups which may easily be seen by research sponsors as The Other. The doctors at Buchenwald and Auschwitz, for example, had little trouble distancing themselves from the pain that they inflicted on subjects in their medical experiments because the subjects were all Other: they were Jews or Poles or homosexuals or Gypsies or Slavs or mental patients, and especially important, they were all prisoners, they all had tatoos, and their heads had all been shaved. They did not look like "Us," and they did not act like "Us." It was easy, though of course not morally justified, for doctors to perceive the prisoner-subjects as The Other.

I do not wish at all to hint, not even indirectly, that today's research sponsors of HIV vaccine trials are somehow like the Nazi doctors. Today's vaccine researchers are highly compassionate and are not racially prejudiced as were the doctors of the Third Reich who worked in Auschwitz and Buchenwald and Birkenau. No one who has seen the effects of the pandemic in Uganda or Rwanda or any of the other hardest hit nations could fail to be greatly moved by the deep tragedy of it, and by the powerful sufferings of whole families and whole regions. What I do wish to underscore, though, is how easy it is for ordinary human beings to feel differently toward The Other than we feel toward someone whom we perceive as Us. Whenever we perceive someone as Other we become less likely to understand them, and even less likely to make an effort to understand them. We are less likely to take their sufferings and their burdens as seriously as we take the sufferings and burdens of people whom we perceive as Us. I am inclined to think that this tendency in us weak and ignorant human beings is a rather prevalent tendency, but it is certainly not a good one. It stems from a weakness and a narrowness of perception, and we have a strong moral obligation to strive to overcome it. We must strive to appreciate the sufferings and burdens of others as much as we appreciate the sufferings and burdens in our own lives. Research sponsors particularly should take very seriously the insight of Mrs Eva Mozes-Kor.

Eva is still alive. She and her twin sister Miriam were human subjects in Dr Josef Mengele's experiments on twins, at Birkenau.

> To look back at my childhood is to remember my experiences as a human guinea pig in the Birkenau laboratory of Dr Josef Mengele. To recount such painful memories is to relive the horrors of human experimentation, where people were used as merely objects or means to a scientific end.[1]

Mrs Mozes-Kor proceeds to describe the horror of these experiments in which she and her sister were subjects, some of which involved studies in genetics and some of which concerned germ warfare, and how they were conducted. Interested readers can find and read (in the book cited below) her moving six page account of what it was like to be one of those twins, but for our purposes here I want to focus on her conclusions.

> I hope that what was done to me will never again happen to another human being. This is the reason I have told my painful story. Those who do research must be compelled to obey international law. Scientists should continue to do research. But if a human being is ever used in the experiments, the scientists must make a moral commitment never to violate a person's human rights and human dignity. The scientist must respect the wishes of the subjects. Every time scientists are involved in human experimentation, they should try to put themselves in the place of the subject and see how they would feel. The

> scientists of the world must remember that the research is being done for the sake of mankind and not for the sake of science; scientists must never detach themselves from the humans they serve. I hope with all my heart that our sad stories will in some special way impel the international community to devise laws and rules to govern human experimentation.[2]

We will examine later in this book a document, sponsored and published by the Council for International Organizations of Medical Sciences (CIOMS) and the World Health Organization, titled *International Ethical Guidelines for Biomedical Research Involving Human Subjects*, published in its final form in late 1993, after long years of consultation and research. We will be exploring this document in detail, but for now it would be well to consider Eva's key words: "Every time scientists are involved in human experimentation, they should try to put themselves in the place of the subject and see how they would feel."

I again wish to emphasize that the human experiments performed by the Nazi doctors in the concentration camps are not here being compared to today's HIV vaccine trials. These are two entirely different categories of human experiments. The former were done with utter disregard for human beings and human suffering, and the latter are being planned by compassionate researchers with the greatest concern for the well being of humanity in general, and the research subjects in particular. The only similarity is that both involve the participation of human beings as research subjects, and whenever human beings participate as volunteers in research protocols, there is some degree of risk that they will be seen more as a means than as ends, more as an Other than as an Us. Eva's words are reminders to us to overcome this tendency to see other human beings as Other, particularly when those others look and act differently than we do. Eva asks us to "put ourselves in the place of," particularly when it comes to medical research involving human subjects.

The unspoken conclusion to Eva's words is a variation on the Golden Rule (to do unto others as you would have others do unto you). The variation, sometimes called the Silver Rule, is phrased thus: do not do unto others what you would not wish others to do unto you.[3] This is Eva's main request to researchers: put yourself in place of the Other. Anticipate the Other's concerns. Do not do to them what you would not wish done to you. If ever any principle should be kept foremost in the minds of those who undertake human subjects research, this is that principle.

Now let us consider, from the perspective of the Antithesis position, some of the potential hazards, large and small, more probable and less probable, that may have to be borne by those who would choose to volunteer in these vaccine trials.

11.1 NO FUTURE PROTOCOLS

The opportunity to participate in a future vaccine research protocol is, in all likelihood, effectively sacrificed when one volunteers for these present experiments. Should a more promising candidate vaccine be developed in the future – and future candidate vaccines would almost certainly be in some ways superior – today's volunteers would be excluded from participating in that research.[4] Reasons for exclusion might vary, but would probably be built around the notion that these subjects had been "contaminated" by another significant variable, viz., exposure to a previous vaccine. Volunteers in today's experiments should know that they will probably not be able to participate in future vaccine research. This should be considered a "harm" for them, but (in my opinion) perhaps not the most important one. That this "harm" would actually happen to subjects in the present studies is a virtual certainty.

11.2 IMMEDIATE SYSTEMIC REACTIONS

A usually mild, but still real, systemic reaction sometimes immediately follows upon a vaccination procedure. Sometimes the reaction is as mild as a headache, local pain at the site of the injection, and a fever, but sometimes the reaction can be more severe, including symptoms as serious as convulsions. Subjects will want to be aware of these possibilities.

11.3 POTENTIAL IMMUNE TOLERANCE

The possibility exists, though it may be a relatively small one, that a subject who receives this present candidate vaccine could become immune to the effects of any future HIV vaccines. This circumstance, if it were to come about, would be called "immune tolerance" and would have the effect of rendering a person

> immunologically unresponsive to the original antigen [HIV], i.e., viral protein(s) capable of inducing immune responses. Immune tolerance may prevent the immune system from mounting any response upon "seeing" this antigen again.[5]

No one presently knows how likely or unlikely this occurrence might be, nor will they know until phase III trials are well under way, but it is within the realm of possibility.[6]

If this were to occur it would have two serious consequences: a) It would mean that this person's immune system would no longer mount any response at all against HIV. It would mean that if this person were to become infected with HIV, the immune system would not fight the virus at all, so progression to disease would likely be more rapid than normal. b) Immune tolerance would also mean that if an effective vaccine against HIV were to be developed and proven successful at some time in the future, this volunteer would not be able to use it because they would not respond to it at all. It would do them no good. They would probably not even be offered a future successful vaccine, especially if it is a vaccine of the whole attenuated virus type, for fear that it would simply infect the person and cause them to develop AIDS.

This risk, though perhaps small, may be a significant one in the minds of some potential volunteers.

11.4 ENHANCED INFECTIVITY

A more important hazard for volunteers is the uncertain possibility of "antibody enhanced infectivity."

> It has been shown by a number of investigators that some HIV antibodies actually help HIV enter host cells, primarily

monocyte cells. This phenomenon is called antibody enhanced infectivity. Antibodies that enhance HIV infectivity have been identified in the serum of HIV-infected patients and in HIV infected and immunized animals.[7]

This potential hazard would mean that subjects inoculated with the candidate vaccine could actually be at *greater* risk for disease than non-vaccinated persons.[8] It would mean that persons who have developed antibodies to HIV (which is what most vaccines stimulate the body to do), and who then subsequently became exposed to HIV through one of the usual routes of infection (which is what phase III subjects will be doing), would then be

1 more likely to become infected (i.e., more *easily* infected) with the virus,
2 more likely to progress to disease,
3 more likely to progress to disease faster, and/or
4 perhaps more likely to develop a more serious form of disease than non-vaccinated persons.

Antibody-enhanced infectivity in candidate viral vaccines is not, unfortunately, either unknown or unprecedented. According to studies cited below, the phenomenon has been shown to exist in at least three or four candidate vaccines for various viral diseases. This hazard became enough of a danger that it blocked research into a vaccine against respiratory syncytial virus (RSV, the major cause of infantile pneumonia) thirty years ago. When an RSV vaccine was undergoing testing in infants in the 1960s "researchers found to their surprise that a strong immune response against the virus can, for unknown reasons, actually enhance the disease."[9] Research was stopped because the hazard was considered too great a risk for the subjects in the trials. This candidate RSV vaccine had already been through phase I and II trials and had been "shown to be nontoxic and antigenic in adult volunteers and nontoxic in infants and children before the larger efficacy study was initiated. The apparent sensitizing effect of the vaccine was entirely unexpected."[10]

The problem of antibody enhanced infectivity has also "been shown to be important in other viral diseases such as dengue fever and rabies."[11] It was a problem in some earlier measles vaccines as well.[12]

I believe this risk, if it is indeed as real as the literature suggests, is a significant one. Subjects in phase III trials may have the experience of the subjects in phase I and II trials to give them some estimate of the likelihood of this occurrence, but perhaps not (as we have just seen with the RSV experimental vaccine). The number of subjects in phase I and II trials may simply be too small to demonstrate the risk, or the length of the trials too short (only one or two years) to establish just how serious or likely this risk actually is. Or the subjects in phase I and II trials may simply be at too low a risk to demonstrate the enhancement that would occur only in the presence of encounter with wild virus. In any case, subjects in phase III trials will probably have no more information on what level of risk to expect for antibody-enhanced infectivity than we have right now. (The problem of enhanced infectivity with the measles vaccine mentioned above was not discovered to be a significant problem until long after phase I and II trials had been completed, and the vaccine had already been administered to "hundreds of thousands of recipients."[13]) In sum, the risk for antibody-enhanced infectivity in HIV vaccines may be fairly high or not very high. We simply do not yet know.[14] And unfortunately we cannot know until we test the candidate vaccines in human populations.[15]

I imagine that some volunteers will see this risk as important enough to decline participation in the trials. When it is made clear to them that "antibody-dependent enhancement of HIV is [truly] a genuine concern,"[16] they may conclude that this risk alone offsets the potential (perhaps small potential) for protection against HIV infection offered by the vaccine. All potential volunteers should be made to fully understand this potential hazard.

11.5 DISCRIMINATION

11.5.1 The Problem

Social discrimination due to the volunteers' new HIV antibody status should be expected.[17] Perhaps for many years these volunteers will be HIV antibody positive (HIVAb+) as a result of being given an HIV vaccine. They may find that when they wish to donate blood or other organs or tissues, or enlist in military service, or apply for health or life insurance, or travel internationally, or even be treated by certain health care or dental practitioners, that they are subjected to unfair discrimination. They may be treated with hostility by neighbors, friends, or work associates. They may have difficulties finding a marriage partner.

> The potential for harm to one's personal reputation also comes with trial participation. The peers of potential participants may view cooperating with government researchers as evidence of gullibility or foolhardy complicity with authority. Participants should know that such social discrimination could seriously affect their everyday lives and may not be compensable.[18]

Moreover, the degree of social discrimination faced by volunteers in phase III trials is liable to be significantly higher than the risk of discrimination faced by those in phase I and II trials, since most of the subjects in phase I, and many of the subjects in phase II trials, will probably be from the middle classes of a society and will also be from groups at lower risk of infection.

Already, even before trials begin, the social discrimination suffered by persons who are HIV+ is severe. In Thailand, for example, it is reported that one of the biggest problems facing HIV+ persons is the social discrimination leveled against them. "Disclosure of a positive status," says one account, "usually leads to the loss of employment, isolation from the community, and problems within the family."[19] It may lead to numerous other problems as well. And we can be sure that the fear of HIV+ persons is not unique to Thailand.

Researchers will probably provide each volunteer with official documentation certifying that their HIVAb+ status is due to their participation in a vaccine trial, and will probably also provide a toll-free phone line for doubters to call and confirm.[20] Researchers will probably also make pre-arrangements with insurance companies and other agencies so they will accept such documents, unless there are extenuating circumstances. But there may be good reason to doubt that these documents would ever be taken seriously. In the first place, documents can be forged and phone numbers can be bogus, so an effective method of insuring authenticity would need to be devised. But more importantly, the persons to whom you would present such documents might not accept them because they may be secretly thinking, "Of course I see that you were in a vaccine experiment a few years ago, and that caused you to become HIVAb+, even though you were not infected with the virus. But perhaps you have also become infected with the real virus in the interval since that vaccine experiment, and I have no simple and quick way of testing for that. Also, I wonder if the researchers might have chosen you to participate in their vaccine trials because you are a person who is at higher than normal risk for HIV infection.[21] So I think I'll just play it safe and not hire you, not let you join the army, not let you donate blood, not sell you our insurance, not etc. etc."

This hypothetical person's thinking is not illogical, since the volunteer could very well have become really infected with the virus since participation in the vaccine experiment. In fact, it would be a safe bet that the volunteer probably has engaged in some risky behaviors. As we will see below, most volunteers would not have been chosen as subjects in the vaccine trials if the researchers did not have good reason to believe that they would in some manner expose themselves to the virus now and then. Phase III vaccine trials must, after all, be done with subjects who are at some significant risk of exposure to the virus, otherwise the research would be pointless. Thus, our hypothetical secret thinker is correct in reasoning that this candidate is probably a person who is, or who was, at some fairly high risk of becoming HIV infected. In any event, whether we consider this thinking to be correct or not, it is very likely that this sort of thinking will occur, viz., thinking which leads to discrimination against volunteers.

It is indeed reasonable to assume that such real discrimination will occur at some times in that volunteer's future life. In fact any interested reader can peruse some first person accounts of real discrimination against HIV+ persons who live in developing nations. Richardson and Bolle have collected a wide variety of such personal interviews in their book titled *Wise Before Their Time.*[22] Some persons have even been socially stigmatized by their mere association with an "AIDS" trial,[23] and the potential for such discrimination is unlikely to diminish.

In order to help minimize such social discrimination, research sponsors should provide volunteers with all the protections they can offer, including certificates, toll free phone numbers for confirmation, and free ELISA and Western Blot tests for HIV antibodies for as many years as necessary. Unfortunately, according to one study, in up to 40 per cent of vaccine trial volunteers, even the more specific Western Blot test will be unable to distinguish between a positive test that is due to receiving a vaccine, and a positive test that is due to being actually infected with HIV.[24] This means that, even with the tests presently used to determine whether a subject is *actually* HIV+, or just *appears to be* HIV+ because of having received a vaccine, up to 40 per cent of volunteers could be mis-identified as actually infected with HIV, using both of today's standard HIV tests, the ELISA and the Western Blot. More complex candidate vaccines are already being proposed for new studies, vaccines in which it will be even more difficult to distinguish apparent HIV infection from actual HIV infection.[25]

There are viral detection methods, such as antigen capture assay, viral culture and the PCR test,[26] however, which test for the presence of the actual virus, rather than just for the presence of antibodies to the virus. These methods are able to distinguish between a vaccine-induced positive response, and an infection-induced positive response. Unfortunately, these methods are more expensive and require some degree of laboratory sophistication and may, therefore, not be as readily available in developing nations.[27] If possible, however, some sort of free viral detection method should also be made available to volunteers for as long as necessary.[28] Free intervention services and/or legal services in the event of discrimination should also be provided to all subjects.

These are some of the precautions that trial sponsors will probably provide to their volunteers. But volunteers should also be made aware of the very real likelihood that in their future lives they will probably suffer some forms of discrimination, and that some of these acts of discrimination (e.g., in hiring or firing, in housing, in blood and organ donations, in application for military service, in application for some kinds of jobs, in application for insurance,[29] for travel visas, and etc.) will not be resolved in the volunteer's favor. Persons seeking travel visas to Russia, for example, may at some point be required to be tested for HIV. Any applicants who test positive would simply not be granted entry visas.[30]

Volunteers who live in developing nations face additional struggles. In many cultures a right to privacy and to confidentiality about personal medical information has not been as strongly established as in some industrial nations. (Although not typical, in some regions of China, for example, there is sometimes public posting in medical clinics of "highly personal information about individuals' health status, inoculations, women's menstrual cycles, and other data."[31])

In addition, it will probably be commonly known in many communities who the people are who are participating in these vaccine trials; or at least it may be easily discovered who they are. Some community members might easily make uncomplimentary assumptions about persons who volunteer for HIV trials: people might assume that these volunteers had been "dirtied" by the vaccine, or that they had been infected by it, or that they had been chosen as a volunteer because they were at high risk for infection, and so on.[32] And additionally for those subjects who do become infected with the virus during the course of the trials, it may be (in some close-knit communities) very easily discovered who got infected and who did not. Those infected persons can expect potentially serious discrimination.

Nor is HIV serostatus the only information that is potentially sensitive for subjects. Drug use practices, types and frequency of sexual practices, and identity and/or number of sexual partners are all equally sensitive information, and if volunteers are not confident that such information will be kept private, they may be reluctant to participate in a trial which will require them to disclose such information to researchers.

11.5.2 Confidentiality: Relativism vs Essentialism

Furthermore, it may be that confidentiality and privacy are not values at all in some communities. In those communities, then, researchers and public health officials would be faced with a serious meta-ethical issue: should they impose strict confidentiality standards on the community in order to protect the welfare of the volunteers, even though confidentiality and privacy do not have a place in the values of that community? Or should sponsors simply accept the prevalent standards of the community and not act to protect the privacy of individual volunteers? Should a value such as "the right to privacy," which might be perceived in that community as a "western world" value, be simply imposed on the community in order to protect individual subjects, or should the privacy of the individuals be ignored in order to respect the ethos of the community? How should this question be resolved?

This question is sometimes referred to as the thorny question of "medical-ethical imperialism." If you answer the question in one way, and say "Yes, the value of protecting individual volunteers is so important that it must be provided for even though the prevailing standards of that community do not endorse the value of the individual's right to privacy," then you risk being labeled a medical-ethical imperialist. If on the other hand you say "No, the value of respecting the local community standards is so important that we will not impose the value of privacy and confidentiality, even though in many parts of the world (and in the WHO/CIOMS *Guidelines*) privacy is seen as a significant human right," then you run the risk of simply running roughshod over the personal safety of the individual volunteers in that community.[33]

At the root of this issue is an even more basic philosophical question about the universalizability of ethical norms. I call it the conflict between ethical relativism and ethical essentialism. The position of ethical relativism holds that no values are universal and hence that no values hold true absolutely, always and everywhere. Ethical relativism sees that different communities do empirically have different ethical norms, and it concludes from this observation that therefore these communities also ethically have the moral right to have whatever norms they choose.

Ethical essentialism, on the other hand, holds that not all values or actions are equally valid or worthy. Ethical essentialism holds that some acts are wrong, even if there is a whole community that endorses them. Ethical essentialism would hold, for example, that torture is wrong, that slavery is wrong, and that genocide is wrong, even though whole communities might endorse those practices and live by them. Ethical essentialism holds that some acts are essentially, in themselves, in their essence, wrong, and should not be endorsed by anyone or any community.

This issue is most complex and multifaceted. Some philosophers argue that the tension between these two positions is *the* defining ethical issue in any modern pluralistic democracy; others have even claimed that this tension is the key philosophic issue that defines what modernity means. The issue is indeed a thorny one, and much too complicated to deal with inside the scope of this small book. And yet, as is the case with many philosophical questions, the way the issue gets decided will have tremendous practical consequences.

In the case we are discussing here, for example, the practical consequence will be either that regulations protecting the confidentiality and privacy of volunteers will be enacted and enforced, or they will not be. What position does the WHO/CIOMS *International Ethical Guidelines* take on the question?

The Council for International Organizations of Medical Sciences, in collaboration with the World Health Organization, which drafted the *International Ethical Guidelines for Biomedical Research Involving Human Subjects*, was sensitive to the issue of medical-ethical imperialism and took steps to insure that they would respect the values of the world's wide variety of cultures. The committee which prepared the document – over more than a decade of research and consultation – was composed of nearly 150 participants from 35 diverse countries. Participants came from both developed and developing countries, "including representatives of ministries of health and medical and other health-related disciplines, health policy-makers, ethicists, philosophers and lawyers."[34]

Representatives attended from all over the world, including some from sub-Saharan Africa, from Asia and from South America (including one representative each from Thailand and Brazil, two of the countries in which WHO plans to initiate phase III HIV vaccine trials; Uganda was not represented, nor was Rwanda nor Tanzania, but Kenya was). After the last conference ended in February of 1992, the *Guidelines* were then revised using all the research, discussions and position papers that had been presented by participants. It was then sent out to the 150 participants for final comments. Dr Bankowski, chair of the committee, explains the process:

> The draft guidelines were revised to reflect the consensus of the conference, but with due regard to minority points of view. The revised draft was then sent for comment to the conference participants, to international associations, and to medical research councils and other interested bodies and institutions in both developed and developing countries. The final text duly reflects the comments received. It has been endorsed by the WHO Global Advisory Committee on Health Research and the Executive Committee of CIOMS, which have recommended its publication and wide distribution.[35]

I mention all this to make it clear that the WHO/CIOMS Committee which drafted these *Guidelines* and published them in 1993 did not act hastily. Committee members made every attempt to face the complex issue of medical-ethical imperialism and to deal with its difficulties as fairly as they could. In the end, however, they had to come down on one side or the other of the question of privacy and confidentiality for research volunteers.

The document they finally published, *International Ethical Guidelines for Biomedical Research Involving Human Subjects,* comes out clearly in favor of supporting and even requiring the protection of confidentiality. It insists that all research subjects have the right to confidentiality concerning their serostatus, their medical records, and even confidentiality as to whether they are participants in the study or not.[36] This message is stated very clearly in the CIOMS *Guidelines.*

11.5.3 Weak Protections for Confidentiality

However, although this document clearly supports the policy of protecting confidentiality, it also recognizes that there are very real *de facto* limitations on that policy, and that these limitations could severely weaken any significant implementation of the policy. Guideline 12 of that document, which addresses the issue of safeguarding confidentiality, states:

> The investigator must establish secure safeguards of the confidentiality of research data. [However,] subjects should be told of the *limits* to the investigators' ability to safeguard confidentiality and of the anticipated consequences of breaches of confidentiality.[37]

This general principle is indeed important, but it should also be made clear to prospective subjects that the "limits to the investigator's ability to safeguard confidentiality" may be very grave, and they should not be minimized. Some jurisdictions, for example, will probably require mandatory reporting of HIVAb+ persons. Trial sponsors, of course, will seek exemptions from such reporting requirements, but if they are not able to acquire such exemptions, prospective volunteers will need to be aware that their confidentiality would probably be seriously compromised if they chose to join the trial.

Even in jurisdictions which do not require mandatory HIVAb+ reporting, protections for confidentiality are often not very strong. One serious instance, to mention only one, of having ineffective safeguards for the protection of subjects' confidentiality, concerns the usual manner of protecting confidential medical records. The usual method of protecting the privacy of these personal documents is simply to require that the individual subject sign a consent form before releasing any confidential medical information. This method, though valuable in many circumstances, does have serious limitations: a) One limitation is that the policy makes it clear to everyone that such records do already exist, and it specifies where they exist and who is the custodian of the records. Clever people with strong motivation will perhaps be able to obtain some of the information they want without getting anyone's formal consent. b) Another limitation on this method of protecting privacy is that great social and personal pressure can be brought to bear on an individual volunteer to sign a release form. c) A third serious limitation on this method of protection is that refusal by a volunteer to give consent for release of information may well be considered damning in itself, much as invocation of Fifth Amendment rights by someone testifying in a trial in the US makes people suspicious that the testifier probably has something to hide. This suspicion alone could lead to acts that would discriminate against the volunteer.

This is all to say that protecting volunteers from discrimination by protecting the privacy of their medical records might be only partially effective.

Another method of protecting against discrimination is to enact laws that proscribe discrimination. Such laws, as everyone knows, can sometimes be extremely difficult to enact and even more difficult to enforce. Witness, for example, the difficulty of enacting and enforcing civil rights legislation in the southern states in the US during the early 1960s, and the violently heated confrontations that have accompanied attempts at gay rights legislation in the US in recent years. Laws protecting civil liberties are sometimes difficult to enact even in the best circumstances of relative civil order, but they can be especially difficult to enact in situations of unstable social order, or if the proposed laws do not really represent the community's actual standards and beliefs. If laws protecting individual rights are enacted in such circumstances, they will probably be exceedingly difficult to enforce. Nevertheless, it is probably better to have such laws on the books than to not have them at all.

A third method of dealing with discrimination is to in some way compensate its victims. (See Chapter 13 below, Compensating Volunteers for Injury.) This of course does not prevent discrimination, nor can any compensation ever replace the individual's actual loss. Furthermore, it might be questionable whether it is even realistic to expect that compensation will actually be given in most cases.

To sum up this section: a person's participation in HIV vaccine trials carries "significant . . . risk of social discrimination or harm."[39] Volunteers should be "apprised in advance of those situations in which trial sponsors might be required to disclose confidential information,"[40] and should be fully informed about the extent and implications of this risk.

11.6 WHOLE VIRUS VACCINES

Vaccines come in three basic forms: killed virus vaccines,[41] live, attentuated virus vaccines, and subunit vaccines. Each type of vaccine uses a slightly different method of stimulating an immune response.[42] The first two types, if used against HIV, would carry significantly more risk than subunit vaccines.

11.6.1 Inactivated Virus Vaccines

A killed or inactivated virus vaccine uses the whole virus, minus the genetic material in its core, to stimulate a successful immune response. (Pseudovirion vaccines are genetically engineered virus-like particles which closely resemble a live three dimensional virus, but also have no genetic material in their core.) Inactivated virus vaccines have been used successfully against rabies, influenza, and polio (Salk vaccine).[43] These vaccines do stimulate an immune response, but the risk is that the process used to inactivate the viruses may have been imperfect and not all viruses got killed. If this happened while using a killed virus vaccine for HIV, then some persons in the vaccine trials would be accidentally injected with an active virus, and hence may become infected with HIV and progress to AIDS. That, of course, would be an important risk.

Such a tragedy did actually occur at one point with the Salk polio vaccine, an inactivated virus vaccine, shortly after the conclusion of the efficacy trials for that vaccine, in 1954.

> Of the 400,000 people inoculated with certain preparations, 79 contracted polio. Another 125 individuals became infected through contact with those vaccinated. Three-quarters of these cases involved paralysis and 11 cases were fatal.[44]

This tragic event, widely known as the Cutter incident, gave warning to all vaccine researchers of the possible consequences that could result if not all viruses had been completely inactivated.

11.6.2 Live, Attenuated Virus Vaccines

A live, attenuated virus vaccine uses active viruses, but viruses which have been in some way weakened. Many of the vaccines currently in use against viral diseases are of the live, attenuated form, including the Sabin oral polio vaccine, and the vaccines for measles, yellow fever and mumps[45]. The advantage of using attenuated virus vaccines is that the virus continues to exist in the vaccinee's body, continues to replicate, and therefore continues to stimulate an immune response as long as the person lives.

> Attenuated viruses continue to reproduce, thereby acting as a constant source of antigenic stimulus to the immune system. Thus attenuated vaccines appear to provide lifelong immunity without requiring periodic boosters.[46]

Thus, the advantage of attenuated virus vaccines is that they could theoretically continue to protect persons against disease for the remainder of their lives. For this reason alone an attenuated virus vaccine for HIV would be extremely desirable.

The risks, however, of using an attenuated virus vaccine for HIV are very high. One of the risks of vaccinating people with a weakened form of HIV is that, since HIV replicates and mutates so rapidly, it would simply eventually mutate back into a highly virulent form.[47] It would, after all, have the rest of the person's life to so mutate. Then all we would have done is infect volunteers with real HIV. (With this form of vaccination, the attenuated virus particles could also be transmissible to others via blood and body fluids, which may be beneficial, if the vaccine is safe, but may be deadly if it is not.)

Such mutations that revert to virulence are by no means unknown. The Sabin oral polio vaccine, for example, is an attenuated virus vaccine and it does happen, even with that extremely safe vaccine, that in very rare cases (one in every two or three million vaccinations) the attenuated virus will mutate back to its virulent form within the body of the vaccinated person and cause a case of active paralytic poliomyelitis.[48] Also, in present SIV vaccine studies, a recent study in the UK using an attenuated SIV vaccine in rhesus macaque monkeys, resulted in the attenuated virus actually reverting, over a rather short time, back to a virulent form and causing one monkey to come down with simian AIDS.[49]

With HIV, which is so highly and rapidly mutable, this risk is serious; so serious, in fact, that I know of only one candidate HIV vaccine in development now that is of the attenuated form, and it has not reached even phase I trials.[50] Many doubt that it ever will. Researchers recognize that one of HIV's most successful attributes is its ability to replicate rapidly and mutate often. Whether it would mutate toward greater virulence or toward lesser virulence is anybody's guess.[51] Evidence so far, however, seems to overwhelmingly indicate that, in an environment with relatively mild selective pressures, HIV generally mutates toward increased virulence.[52]

Another problem with attenuated virus vaccines is that they pose additional risks to persons who are in any way immunocompromised.[53] Such persons, because of their suppressed immune systems, may be overwhelmed even by a weakened form of the pathogen against which they are being vaccinated. In some lesser developed communities, of course, malnutrition may contribute to some cases of immunosuppression. Undetected HIV disease may also put persons at risk for immunosuppression. Any persons or groups who may be immunosuppressed for any of these reasons would probably need to be tested for immunocompetence before administering a live virus vaccine to them. This would require screening those populations for various markers of immunosuppression before administering a live virus vaccine that might put them at serious risk. Such large scale screening would add one more enormous logistical challenge to an already complex set of logistical difficulties, when it came time to actually deploy a successful HIV vaccine.

11.6.3 Subunit Vaccines

Subunit vaccines are not made from whole live viruses, nor from killed viruses, but from certain key fragments of the virus, often surface proteins. In these first generation HIV-1 vaccines, the subunit that has been most often used is the glycoprotein gp120 (or its precursor, gp160),[54] which is the portion of the viral surface that actually binds to the CD4 molecule on the surface of human cells. Sometimes a viral core protein, such as p17, may be used instead.[55] Often, chemical or biological adjuvants are injected (or ingested) along with the vaccine in order to help the immune system detect the subunit, "thereby producing a more potent immune response".[56]

Subunit vaccines can be developed in three different forms. In one form, a) the subunits themselves are simply grown in vitro (e.g., in ovarian cells of Chinese hamsters), collected, and then injected directly into the vaccinee. In another form, b) a peptide of the subunit – i.e., a subunit of the subunit – is developed and injected into the vaccinee. And in a third form, c) the gene that encodes for that particular subunit is taken from the DNA stage of HIV replication and spliced into the DNA of another virus, a vector virus such as vaccinia or canary pox virus. Then the newly engineered vector is injected into the vaccinee, and when that vector virus replicates in his or her cells, it will express the selected viral subunit for which the gene encodes. The presence of that subunit will then (it is hoped) stimulate an immune response against any wild virus that displays the same subunit. These are called recombinant vector subunit vaccines, and they do actually use a live virus, though it is not the virus which is responsible for the infection that is being vaccinated against.

The advantage of the a) and b) forms of subunit vaccines (the subunit and the peptides) is that they are not whole viruses, so have absolutely no capacity to infect the vaccinee or anyone else the vaccinee may contact. Their primary disadvantage, however, is that they seem to produce an immune response that is specific to only those subtypes and strains of HIV that have the exact same form of the subunit as is in the vaccine (i.e., homologous strains), and the response seems to be relatively short-lived.[57] These would be significant disadvantages. The advantage of the c) form using a vector virus would be that the immune response would probably last much longer, since the vector would continue to replicate inside the vaccinee, would continue to express the desired HIV surface subunit, and hence would continue to stimulate an immune response in the vaccinee as long as it continued to replicate. This would be a significant advantage.

The disadvantage of the c) form, however, is that it requires the introduction of a live, albeit usually harmless, virus into persons who may be immunocompromised already and not in good enough condition to fight off yet another virus. There have purportedly been deaths from fulminant vaccinia disease caused by the vaccinia vector virus in some recombinant vaccines for other diseases. Furthermore, besides this risk to the vaccinated individual, there is the additional risk that the process of immunization itself will probably produce purulent sores that could put other nearby immunosuppressed third parties at risk of infection with a disease that they are not capable of fighting off.[58] Deaths from fulminant vaccinia disease, while rare, did sometimes even occur during the years that vaccinia virus was being used as a vaccine against smallpox. As recently as 1968, for example, two decades after the US had seen its last case of smallpox, "15 million persons were vaccinated that year [against smallpox], and because of vaccine complications, 240 required hospitalization, 9 died, and 4 were permanently disabled."[59] Vaccinia virus, then, while a generally safe vector virus, is still potentially a disease-causing agent, and its use in immunocompromised communities may be problematic.

These latter risks, however, seem to be more of a problem for those recombinant vaccines in which vaccinia virus is the vector used for carrying in the subunit gene, and vaccinia is indeed the vector being used in some of the recombinant subunit vaccines presently in phase I and II testing. Vaccinia, after all, is the agent originally responsible for the disease of cowpox. Cowpox is normally quite a mild disease in humans, but we do not yet know the full effects cowpox might have if it were to be introduced into persons who are already immunocompromised. Because of this potential risk, other viruses are also being explored as potential vectors. Avipox virus (canary pox) vector vaccines are just beginning phase I testing. This virus has the peculiar trait of replicating only one time in human host cells, so the infection is actually aborted before it can develop into anything that would cause disease.[60] As Seattle researchers Julie McElrath and Larry Corey point out, the canary pox virus

> can infect avian fibroblasts but induces [only] one round of replication in the human host. Because it causes an abortive infection, the risk of transmission to immunocompromised patients is minimized.[61]

Other vectors that are presently being investigated for potential HIV vaccine use include adenovirus, rhinovirus, BCG (presently used as a tuberculosis vaccine in many parts of the world), *salmonella*, and hepatitis B.[62]

To sum up, then: the advantage of subunit vaccines is that they are almost certainly lower risk vaccines, and in fact are probably the safest of the three kinds of vaccines.

They are also probably the least effective of the vaccine types, because (as we have seen) each vaccine seems to protect against only a very few variants of HIV, viz., those variants that have a gp120 (or 160) molecule which is virtually identical to the gp120 that was used for the vaccine. Furthermore, the immune response stimulated by these subunit vaccines seems to last only several months to two years at the most. This means that revaccination would be necessary quite often.[63] That would be a significant logistical challenge for already overburdened public health services in any community, whether developed or not.

Each of these three types of vaccines, then, has its own virtues and dangers. Volunteers should be made fully aware of the risks involved with the vaccine type they are using. If there is any meaningful risk at all of becoming infected with HIV and developing AIDS, participants will have to weigh that risk against the potential benefits of the vaccine. Becoming infected with HIV and developing AIDS is a harm for which it would be almost impossible to compensate a person.

11.7 BEING MONITORED

Another of the "inconveniences and hazards reasonably to be expected" by vaccine trial participants, particularly in phase III studies, is that they will need to be monitored by researchers for a number of years, perhaps for many years, perhaps for the rest of their lives. In addition to preliminary screening, educating and counseling prior to vaccination, subjects will also need to be tested regularly after vaccination, and be given checkups and counseling regularly, perhaps as often as once every two or three months, or even more often. Checkups, testing and counseling will need to continue for some years, during the entire course of the trial.

How long might phase III trials last? The answer to that question, about when the endpoint of the study would be, depends entirely on the "criterion of effectiveness" in that study. If the criterion of effectiveness in phase III trials is only a) the emergence of certain immune system markers, then that could be achieved in a matter of months, so the trial would be short. This criterion (immunogenicity), however, is applicable in phase II trials only, and would not be an adequate criterion of efficacy for phase III trials by anyone's account.[64] So immune system markers would not be used as a criterion, at least not in these first generation vaccine trials.

If the criterion of effectiveness is prevention of infection, then trials lasting three to five years may be adequate. But if the one of the criteria of effectiveness is prevention of disease (or postponement or amelioration of disease), which is the traditional criterion of effectiveness in most vaccines – and this doubtless will be one of the criteria, especially in the early trials – then phase III trials will need to last much longer. How long will subjects need to be followed before we know they will not get AIDS? Ten or fifteen years? Twenty years? For life?[65]

If participants will need to be followed for that long, that means they will need to be checking in with researchers for that number of years, or for the rest of their lives. This may amount to only an inconvenience for many participants, but it may amount to a genuine hardship for others. Some may find their lives restricted in some significant ways due to this requirement that they be available.[66] Volunteers should be made aware of this requirement and its possible attendant inconveniences and hardships.

11.8 FEELING SAFE

One of the biggest risks for participants in vaccine trials is the danger that they will now feel more secure and protected, as a result of having been "vaccinated," and will thus feel freer to engage in risky behaviors. This is no small risk, especially since it operates below the level of conscious motivations. Researchers must be particularly emphatic when they counsel trial participants to avoid risky behaviors. They must make it clear that the candidate vaccine being tested is not a proven protection against anything, and that in fact participants may be at greater risk of infection than if they had not chosen to participate in the study (due to possible factors such as antibody enhanced infectivity). Counselors must also make it abundantly clear that the study is double-blinded and placebo controlled,[67] which means that a substantial percentage of the volunteers will be receiving a completely inert substance that provides absolutely no protection of any kind.[68] Counseling that makes these facts clear must be thorough and forceful. (Such counseling must also, of course, be culturally and linguistically appropriate.)

In spite of such counseling, however, some subjects may choose to secretly get tested for HIV antibodies in some other testing facility in order to determine whether they were one of the subjects who was lucky enough to get the candidate vaccine. That is, they might choose to "unblind" themselves in the study. This unblinding could have two unfortunate consequences, one for the individuals and one for the study itself: a) the unfortunate consequence for the individual subject is that they may now feel even safer than when they first joined the study and may therefore feel much freer to engage in risky sexual or needle-sharing behaviors. Such behavior change could put that subject at even higher risk of HIV infection than the risk with which they had lived before joining the study. Such increased risk behavior on the part of those who had unblinded themselves might also b) have an unfortunate effect on the statistical structure of the study itself, as explained by one group of researchers:

> If volunteers who discover that they have received the vaccine are falsely reassured and then engage in high-risk behavior at a greater rate than do placebo recipients, a less-than-optimal vaccine candidate (one with an efficacy of 50% to 60%) may be judged completely ineffective because of selective high-risk behavior among decoded vaccine recipients. . . . The unblinding of a few vaccine trial participants has already occurred in phase I trials.[69]

Those who design these trials will want to devise ways of dealing with the problem of unblinding. They will want to be able to a) identify those who are most likely to try to unblind themselves (e.g., by noticing, during pre-trial counseling, that these prospective subjects' main motivation for wanting to join the trial is to be protected by the "vaccine"), so that these persons might not be selected to participate in the trial;[70] b) somehow motivate persons who do join the trial to not want to unblind themselves; c) somehow identify – probably by self-report – those who do unblind themselves, either deliberately or inadvertently; d) provide regular blinded HIV testing for those subjects who are worried that they may have exposed themselves to infection, so that they can be notified if their test is positive for the virus (not just for antibodies to the virus); and e) have open and frank discussion about some of the consequences of unblinding.

In addition, some trial subgroups, such as commercial sex workers and injection drug users, may be more likely than most to be arrested, charged with a crime, and incarcerated. It is not unusual for penal systems to require mandatory HIV screening for all inmates, so it is not unlikely that the problem of unblinding will be a very real one in these trials, even if it only happens inadvertently.[71] Possible consequences for the statistical significance of the trials will need to be determined.

Probably the best way to minimize the likelihood of such untoward consequences is to insure that counseling about the risks of the study is thorough and clear, that subjects are made fully aware that this candidate vaccine is only *possibly* effective, that even if it is effective in some persons it may be completely ineffective in others, and that it must not be relied on at all for protection against anything. In fact, in some cases,

> even vaccines that produce very good immunity may be overwhelmed by vast numbers of invading organisms and a "breakthrough" infection may result. This is not uncommonly seen, for example, with measles vaccination in developing countries where "breakthrough" infections occur quite frequently in the overcrowded conditions of socio-economically deprived communities, even though the vaccine itself usually provides excellent immunity.[72]

Counseling that makes subjects aware of these realities may be effective in discouraging the feeling that volunteers in the study are somehow safer and can engage in risky behaviors.

Furthermore, in addition to the verbal counseling, condoms should probably also be provided free of charge to all participants, and depending on the setting of the study and the populations being studied, clean needles for drug injection should perhaps be provided as well.[73]

Research sponsors must be particularly cognizant of their obligation to observe one of the most basic principles of medical ethics: "first do no harm" (*primum non nocere*). This means: at least don't make things worse. In vaccine trials that use killed virus vaccines or attenuated virus vaccines, there could be, as we saw above, some additional risk that participants may accidentally receive a vaccine with virus in it that is capable of causing disease. If this were to happen, then the vaccine trial would have made things worse for those particular subjects. Furthermore, if this tragic accident were to come to pass, and these trial participants continued to engage in risky behaviors (unprotected sex, sharing needles, etc), then they would be putting not only themselves at risk, but they would be spreading to others the virus with which they had been accidentally infected. Vaccine trial participants would, in that case, be worsening the spread of the epidemic, and trial sponsors would bear some of the responsibility for that.

For all these reasons, there is a strong duty to provide clear, thorough and effective counseling to all participants. (See Chapter 12 below for the ethical problem of counseling with dual intent.)

11.9 IMMUNOSUPPRESSION

Another danger, even of the safer gp 120 subunit vaccines, is that the vaccine itself could have a compromising effect on the immune system of the vaccinated person. Two mechanisms for such immunocompromise may occur, syncytia and decrease in CD4 availability.

1 Syncytia is the pathological bunching together of a cluster of individual T4 cells into one big clump. All the T4 cells in the clump are disabled, and therefore become ineffective in their role as chief directing cell in the overall immune system response. The causes of syncytia (from the Greek: syn = together, and cyt = cell) are not entirely clear, but seem to be related to the function of gp120 and its ability to bind to the CD4 molecule on T4 cells. Whatever the mechanism of the pathology, the result is a compromise in the overall functioning of the person's immune system.[74]

2 A second possible mechanism of immunosuppression could be a decrease in the number of CD4 molecules available on the surface of T4 cells for performing their normal functions. Dr Barry Shoub, Director of the National Institute of Virology at the University of Witwatersrand in Johannesburg, explains:

> Another difficulty with the use of gp120 as an antigen in a vaccine is the fact that its attachment to the CD4 receptor may compete with the physiological function where the macrophage attaches to the CD4 receptor of the [T4] lymphocyte to present new antigens to the immune system. An additional fear is the fact that the antibodies elicited by gp120 could attach to the surface proteins of the macrophage involved in this interaction with the CD4 antigen.[75]

If either of these two developments did occur then the vaccinees' normal immune response would be compromised to some degree. This means that trial subjects would thus be more susceptible to opportunistic infections which would take advantage of their weakened immune response.

11.10 AUTOIMMUNITY

Autoimmune disorders are those in which the immune system has lost some of its ability to distinguish between self and non-self cells, and consequently begins to attack some of the host's own self cells.

Shoub and others believe that there is some risk that vaccinees could develop autoimmune disorders.[76] If the CD4 function is compromised (as explained just above), or if the antibodies elicited by the vaccine were to attach to the surface proteins of the macrophages that come to dock with the CD4 molecule on the surface of the T4 cells, then there is a risk that the immune system could begin to target the host's own body.[77] Autoimmune disorders can be quite serious, so if this risk is a probable one, potential volunteers will want to be aware of it.

11.11 MALIGNANCIES

HIV unfortunately belongs to the family of viruses (Retroviridae) which have been associated with the development of malignancies. Because of this, if vaccines are made from whole inactivated viruses, or from whole attenuated viruses (but not if they are made from subunits of the virus), there could be some risk of cells developing malignancies. Shoub explains:

> This . . . would make the use of the virus itself unsuitable to develop as an attenuated vaccine . . ., or as a "killed" or inactivated whole virus vaccine (because the nucleic acid would still be present and the genetic information could hold a theoretical danger of being able to transform cells into malignancy).[78]

Shoub seems to indicate that this outcome has not been empirically seen in any work with retroviruses, but that from his knowledge of retroviruses and malignancy, the risk does theoretically exist.[79] What form such a malignancy might take, or what the likelihood is that it would actually develop, is not presently understood.

11.12 NEUROLOGICAL DISEASE OF UNKNOWN ORIGIN

"The most feared situation in any vaccine trial is that cases of severe neurological disease of unknown etiology will be reported among the participants in the first weeks after an injection."[80] A few vaccines currently in use do, though rarely, seem to cause such neurological disorders. A sheep-brain-derived rabies vaccine sometimes (about one per 400 vaccinations) results in myeloencephalitis, and a live attenuated poliovirus vaccine very rarely (about one per one million vaccinations) results in "vaccine paralysis."[81]

In addition, Guillain-Barré syndrome is a well known serious neurologic disorder that very infrequently follows an influenza immunization procedure. A close friend recently suffered a relatively severe attack of the syndrome shortly after receiving his annual influenza vaccine (flu vaccines are made from inactivated viruses). This disease is a demyelinating neuropathy which results in loss of sensation and muscle strength throughout much of the body, particularly the limbs. It has a one to eight per cent fatality rate, but those who do survive it generally recover most of their sensation and muscle strength within six months to a year.

Neuropathies of unknown etiology are an uncommon consequence of some immunization procedures, and the frequency with which they could follow from an HIV vaccine procedure is completely unknown.

To date, there are no tests for determining whether a given vaccine does or does not carry a risk of neuropathy; furthermore, our understanding of the mechanisms by which these neuropathies occur is fairly rudimentary.[82]

11.13 LEARNING YOUR ANTIBODY STATUS

Some have considered the knowledge of their positive antibody status to be a "burdensome knowledge that should not be imposed." A certain number of subjects in these trials (in either a vaccine or placebo arm) will probably become HIV infected in the course of their usual risky behaviors, and when they do, then for them "the necessary surveillance of HIV antibody status might . . . ultimately result in knowledge of HIV infection that the subjects would otherwise have avoided."[83] For some this might not be considered a burden at all, and may even be considered a benefit. But others may consider it a burden imposed on them by their participation in the trial.

11.14 UNKNOWN AND UNANTICIPATED RISKS

In addition to the above risks, some of which may perhaps be known (from phase I and II trials) to have some given degree of likelihood, great or small, there is also the theoretical possibility of completely unanticipated hazards. Birth defects that were the tragic consequence of using Thalidomide were completely unanticipated by researchers and clinicians, and did not show up until years afterwards when some Thalidomide recipients became pregnant and gave birth to severely deformed children.[84]

It is possible that such unanticipated hazards could have shown up earlier in subjects who participated in phase I and phase II trials, but they may not have. Phase I and II trials are typically only one to three years in duration, and typically have only a few hundred subjects, so long term consequences may not come to pass in that shorter time span, in that smaller number of subjects. It may be that some hazards will emerge only in phase III trials, with their larger number of participants and the longer duration of the trials.

There is also the possibility that some unanticipated risks could even affect the regular sex partners of some subjects, thereby putting third parties at risk. This would be ethically analogous to Thalidomide having severe deforming effects on the fetuses of some users, but having no ill effect on the users themselves. This eventuality could potentially increase the number of persons who are at some degree of risk in these trials, and would (if such risks were to actually come to pass) have the consequence of potential increased liabilities for sponsors. This is the problem of endangerment of third parties who have not been informed that they were even at risk, and hence have not been asked for nor given consent to accept such risk.[85] Because of this possibility, research sponsors may want to provide counseling to family and regular partners of subjects who are participating in the trials.

These are some of the risks potentially to be encountered by human subjects in HIV vaccine trials, particularly in developing nations. These risks are real and some are probable. Some of these harms, of course, are clearly more likely to occur than others. For example, not being allowed to participate in future HIV vaccine protocols is very likely to happen; developing immune suppression as a result of a surface subunit vaccine is probably much less likely to occur. Besides the *degree of likelihood* that a given harm will occur, some of these harms are also clearly more *grievous* than others. For example, some forms of social discrimination to which subjects may be vulnerable (loss of jobs, housing, insurance, and etc.) would be much more grievous harms for most people than learning their antibody status.

These are the two dimensions of any potential harm: its likelihood of occurring, and its experienced grievousness if it does occur. Potential harms will probably need to be evaluated in both dimensions. ERCs will probably want to see potential harms evaluated in terms of each of these dimensions, and some subjects may wish to be made aware of such information. (I have proposed the use of some new application forms for detailing the potential harms that prospective subjects may wish to be aware of, and that Ethics Review Committees will definitely want to be aware of when they perform their ethical review of proposed vaccine protocols; these application forms are included as Appendix V in this book.)

Those who hold the Antithesis position insist that volunteers must be made fully aware of all these risks (and perhaps others) before they are asked for their consent to participate in the trials.[86]

NOTES

1. E. Mozes-Kor. "The Mengele Twins and Human Experimentation: A Personal Account." *The Nazi Doctors and the Nuremberg Code: Human Rights in Human Experimentation.* Eds. G. J. Annas and M. A. Grodin (New York, NY: Oxford University Press, 1992) 53–59, p 53.
2. *Ibid.* p 58.
3. This "silver rule can be found in the teachings of virtually all of the world's great spiritual traditions. A few examples: "What you don't want done to yourself, don't do to others" (Confucian, 6th century BC). "Hurt not others with that which pains thyself" (Buddhism, 5th century BC). "Do not do unto others all that which is not well for oneself" (Zoroastrianism, 5th century BC). "Do naught to others which if done to thee would cause thee pain" (Hinduism, Mahabharata, 3d century BC). "What is hateful to yourself, don't do to your fellow man" (Rabbi Hillel, Judaism, first century BC). Etc. from Editor, *The Bulletin of the King County Medical Society*, 73, 12. December (1994) cover.
4. "The first vaccine candidates to be tested in humans are unlikely to be even close to 100% effective, and numerous trials may be necessary." D. Hodel and AIDS Action Foundation Working Group. *HIV Preventive Vaccines: Social, Ethical, and Political Considerations* (AIDS Action Foundation, Office of AIDS Research, National Institutes of Health, 1994), p i.

   Also: "Receiving an ineffective vaccine candidate may render subjects ineligible for future trials." D. Hodel and AIDS Action Foundation Working Group. *HIV Preventive Vaccines: Social, Ethical, and Political Considerations* (AIDS Action Foundation, Office of AIDS Research, National Institutes of Health, 1994), p 27.
5. J. P. Porter, M. J. Glass and W. C. Koff, "Ethical Considerations in AIDS Vaccine Testing," *IRB, A Review of Human Subjects Research,* 11. 3, May–June (1989) 1–4, p 2.
6. "Receiving an ineffective vaccine candidate may render subjects . . . unresponsive to future, more effective vaccines." D. Hodel and AIDS Action Foundation Working Group. *HIV Preventive Vaccines: Social, Ethical, and Political Considerations* (AIDS Action Foundation, Office of AIDS Research, National Institutes of Health, 1994), p 27.
7. G. Stine. *Acquired Immune Deficiency Syndrome: Biological, Medical, Social and Legal Issues.* First ed. (Englewood Cliffs, NJ 07632: Prentice Hall, 1993) 462+xxxii, p 216. Stine cites J. Homsy et al., "The Fe and Not CD4 Receptor Mediates Antibody Enhancement of HIV Infection in Human Cells," *Science,* 244 (1989) 1357–59, and

W. C. Koff, "Development and Testing of AIDS Vaccines," *Science*, 241 (1988) 426–32.

It is not known whether this is a risk with all forms of HIV vaccines, or only with live virus vaccines. See the discussion of the different kinds of vaccines in section 11.6, where the risks of live virus vaccines are discussed. See also *Statement from the Consultation on Criteria for International Testing of Candidate HIV Vaccines* (Geneva: World Health Organization, 1989) 13, p 2.

See also:

> HIV-specific human antibodies can enhance HIV growth in certain types of cultured human cells; several independent research teams using different methodologies have reported reproducible increases of HIV growth in cell cultures in vitro. . . . It is conceivable that vaccine-induced HIV antibodies might be harmful by predisposing to, rather than protecting from, infection and disease. D. S. Burke, "Human HIV Vaccine Trials: Does antibody-dependent enhancement pose a genuine risk?," *Perspectives in Biology and Medicine*, 35, 4 Summer (1992) 511–30, p 511.

8. D. F. Hoth, et al., "HIV Vaccine Development: A Progress Report," *Annals of Internal Medicine*, 8, 7.15 October (1994) 603–11, p 609.
   "[D]isease enhancement due to immunization [is] a serious safety concern." W. N. Rida and D. N. Lawrence, "Some Statistical Issues in HIV Vaccine Trials," *Statistics in Medicine*, 13 (1994) 2155–77, p 2170.
9. J. Cohen, "Bumps on the Vaccine Road," *Science*, 265.2 September (1994) 1371–73, p 1372.
   Consider also: "for example an inactivated respiratory syncytial virus preparation, though apparently innocuous on administration, caused severe complications due to immune enhancement in some young children when they subsequently encountered the wild-type agent." G. L. Ada, "Modern Vaccines," *The Lancet*, 335, March 3 (1990) 523–26, p 526.
   Also: one study demonstrated that the RSV vaccine being studied enhanced viral replication in vaccinated subjects as much as fifty-fold; i.e., RSV replicated in vaccinated subjects fifty times faster than in the non-vaccinated controls. D. S. Burke, "Human HIV Vaccine Trials: Does antibody-dependent enhancement pose a genuine risk?," *Perspectives in Biology and Medicine*, 35, 4 Summer (1992) 511–30, p 521.
10. D. S. Burke, "Human HIV Vaccine Trials: Does antibody-dependent enhancement pose a genuine risk?," *Perspectives in Biology and Medicine*, 35, 4 Summer (1992) 511–30, p 521.
11. B. D. Schoub. *AIDS & HIV in Perspective* (New York, NY: Cambridge University Press, 1994) 268+xx, p 190. Shoub does not make it clear whether this is also a problem in present vaccines for these diseases. We do have a successful inactivated virus vaccine for rabies, of course, so at least in that case the problem was not insoluble.
12. W. N. Rida and D. N. Lawrence, "Some Statistical Issues in HIV Vaccine

Trials," *Statistics in Medicine*, 13 (1994) 2155–77, p 2160. See also D. S. Burke, "Human HIV Vaccine Trials: Does antibody-dependent enhancement pose a genuine risk?," *Perspectives in Biology and Medicine*, 35, 4 Summer (1992) 511–30, p 519–21.

13. D. S. Burke, "Human HIV Vaccine Trials: Does antibody-dependent enhancement pose a genuine risk?," *Perspectives in Biology and Medicine*, 35, 4 Summer (1992) 511–30, p 520–21.

14. Is HIV antibody-dependent enhancement a genuine risk, as it is in human dengue and perhaps respiratory syncytial virus infections, and as it is in animal rabies, feline infectious peritonitis, Aleutian disease, and perhaps other virus infections? Or is HIV enhancement a clinically irrelevant laboratory curiosity, as it seems to be for human yellow fever and Japanese encephalitis virus infections. . . . ? Clearly more information is needed. D. S. Burke, "Human HIV Vaccine Trials: Does antibody-dependent enhancement pose a genuine risk?," *Perspectives in Biology and Medicine*, 35, 4 Summer (1992) 511–30, p 525.

15. Prospective human efficacy trials should be designed to determine whether vaccines confer excess risk, as well as to determine if they confer protection. Special attention must be given to detection of adverse effects of immunization in situations in which enhancement is possible. One such situation could be a vaccine trial conducted in a geographic region where multiple genetically divergent HIV-1 or HIV-2 strains are present. D. S. Burke, "Human HIV Vaccine Trials: Does antibody-dependent enhancement pose a genuine risk?," *Perspectives in Biology and Medicine*, 35, 4 Summer (1992) 511–30, p 526.

16. D. S. Burke, "Human HIV Vaccine Trials: Does antibody-dependent enhancement pose a genuine risk?," *Perspectives in Biology and Medicine*, 35, 4 Summer (1992) 511–30, p 527.

    I have not seen anyone explore the question as to whether there is any risk here to regular sexual or needle-sharing partners of volunteers in these trials. Burke does note that "Passively transferred antibodies [transmitted via blood or via sex?] were also shown to enhance dengue virus growth in vivo experiments in monkeys" (p 519). If such infection-enhancing antibodies could be passed from trial subjects to their sexual or needle-sharing partners, this could constitute a risk to those third parties, and trial sponsors may even have an obligation to see that third parties are made aware of this risk.

    If this risk is real, it could also constitute a significant public health hazard for enhancing the HIV/AIDS pandemic. It would thus be a hazard both to individuals and to the community.

    Furthermore, if Paul Ewald's thesis is correct (and his argument is certainly persuasive), then antibody-enhanced infectivity could have some other disastrous effects as well. It could have the effect of increasing the viral pool, and at the same time increasing the ease of transmission of HIV from one host to another. These two factors would, if the principles of Darwinian medicine are correct, increase the likelihood of HIV mutating toward greater virulence, since there would be fewer selective pressures operating to keep the virus host-friendly.

However, I have seen no discussion of these questions in the literature, perhaps because they are considered to have a low probability. Still, the trials should be designed to monitor for these possible outcomes.

17. Subjects must be apprised of the possibility that they may suffer discrimination as though they were infected with HIV merely because they participate in an HIV vaccine trial. To the extent known, participants should receive full information about possible sources of social discrimination and counseling on how to respond to it.

    The social risks associated with participation in these trials is unprecedented. D. Hodel and AIDS Action Foundation Working Group. *HIV Preventive Vaccines: Social, Ethical, and Political Considerations* (AIDS Action Foundation, Office of AIDS Research, National Institutes of Health, 1994), p 29.
18. D. Hodel and AIDS Action Foundation Working Group. *HIV Preventive Vaccines: Social, Ethical, and Political Considerations* (AIDS Action Foundation, Office of AIDS Research, National Institutes of Health, 1994), p 29.
19. T. Brown and P. Xenos. "AIDS: Epidemic in Asia." *Seattle Post-Intelligencer* October 2, 1994, D1, D3.
20. Subjects should be protected by providing them with "documents attesting to their participation in vaccine trials, or by maintaining a confidential register of trial participants, from which information can be made available to outside agencies at a participant's request." Z. Bankowski, ed. *International Ethical Guidelines for Biomedical Research Involving Human Subjects* (Geneva, Switzerland: Council for International Organizations of Medical Sciences (CIOMS), 1993) 63, p 32.
21. This possibility is clearly delineated in D. F. Hoth, et al., "HIV Vaccine Development: A Progress Report," *Annals of Internal Medicine,* 8, 7.15 October (1994) 603–11, p 609.
22. A. Richardson and D. Bolle, eds. *Wise Before Their Time: People from Around the World Living with AIDS and HIV Tell Their Stories* (London: HarperCollins, 1992) 144.
23. D. Hodel and AIDS Action Foundation Working Group. *HIV Preventive Vaccines: Social, Ethical, and Political Considerations* (AIDS Action Foundation, Office of AIDS Research, National Institutes of Health, 1994), p ii.
24. R. B. Belshe, et al., "Interpreting HIV Serodiagnostic Test Results in the 1990s: Social Risks of HIV Vaccine Studies in Uninfected Volunteers," *Annals of Internal Medicine,* 121, 8.15 October (1994) 584–89, p 584.

    "Moreover, in Africa and other developing countries, the specificity may not be adequate, since some individuals living there may be infected with other viruses that react to the Western blot." W. N. Rida and D. N. Lawrence, "Some Statistical Issues in HIV Vaccine Trials," *Statistics in Medicine,* 13 (1994) 2155–77, p 2161.
25. R. B. Belshe, et al., "Interpreting HIV Serodiagnostic Test Results in

the 1990s: Social Risks of HIV Vaccine Studies in Uninfected Volunteers," *Annals of Internal Medicine,* 121, 8.15 October (1994) 584–89, p 588.

Those vaccinated with BCG vaccine for tuberculosis have the same difficulty: they cannot readily distinguish between a person who tests positive for tuberculosis because they have been vaccinated, and those who test positive because they have been infected with tuberculosis. "Unfortunately... no reliable method can distinguish tuberculin reactions caused by BCG vaccination from those caused by infection with M. tuberculosis." J. R. Starke and K. K. Connelly. "Bacille Calmette-Guérin Vaccine." *Vaccines.* Eds. S. A. Plotkin MD and E. A. Mortimer Jr, MD, second ed. (Philadelphia: W.B. Saunders Company, 1994) 439–73, p 446.

26. Polymerase Chain Reaction (PCR) is a highly sensitive test for the presence of the actual virus, not merely for the presence of antibodies to the virus, as are other HIV screening tests, such as the ELISA and Western blot tests.
27. They also may not solve the problem entirely. Consider: "Even if more definitive tests, such as PCR, are used to detect infection, the problem of misclassification may not be completely solved. HIV mutates readily, and PCR may not detect new mutants." W. N. Rida and D. N. Lawrence, "Some Statistical Issues in HIV Vaccine Trials," *Statistics in Medicine,* 13 (1994) 2155–77, p 2161.
28. The same problem faces BCG vaccinees: the most important laboratory test for the diagnosis of tuberculosis is the mycobacterial culture. Unfortunately, in many poor regions of the world where tuberculosis case rates are high, cultures are not available." J. R. Starke and K. K. Connelly. "Bacille Calmette-Guérin Vaccine." *Vaccines.* Eds. S. A. Plotkin MD and E. A. Mortimer Jr, MD, second ed. (Philadelphia: W. B. Saunders Company, 1994) 439–73, p 447.
29. Research sponsors may even choose to provide independent health insurance for trial volunteers in order to solve this particular problem. This, of course, would raise other problems concerning undue inducement which would need to be clarified and dealt with.
30. S. Efron. "Russia moves toward AIDS tests for foreigners." *Seattle Times* 29 October 1994, A3.
31. G. J. Annas and M. A. Grodin, eds. *The Nazi Doctors and the Nuremberg Code: Human Rights in Human Experimentation* (New York, NY: Oxford University Press, 1992) 371+xxii, p 249.
32. "Anecdotal experience from study nursing staff suggests that once these women [Thai commercial sex workers] abandon prostitution and return to their home villages, they may be stigmatized by study participation and resist attempts for continued follow-up by study staff." B. G. Weniger, "Experience from HIV incidence cohorts in Thailand: implications for HIV vaccine efficacy trials," *AIDS,* 8, 7 (1994) 1007–1010, p 1009.
33. Writing in 1988, well before the 1993 publication of the CIOMS guidelines, Dr Christakis writes:

The straightforward application of ethical standards across cultural barriers is problematic. Confronting AIDS will require rethinking of a narrow, parochial formulation of ethics.

This is not to assert that standards for research ethics should be culturally relative, but rather that they should be culturally relevant. Some ethical standards can and should be met worldwide. An important challenge to Western scientists conducting AIDS vaccine trials is to conform to certain minimum ethical standards regardless of the setting: 1) The trial should be of suitable design and scientific merit; 2) it should involve the free, and where possible, informed consent of the participants; 3) all participants should benefit from proper counseling regarding avoidance of risky behaviors; 4) due consideration should be given to the risks of research participation, using the highest standard of risk/benefit analysis possible; and 5) the countries participating in the study should be allowed fair access to any vaccine arising from the research.

An equally important – and possibly more difficult – challenge to investigators conducting AIDS vaccine trials throughout the world is to be culturally sensitive. . . . Beyond certain minimum standards, there should be tolerance of variability. . . .

What is essential is not that the research meet the same ethical standard worldwide. What is essential is that the research manifest a culturally sensitive and ethically sophisticated concern for the wellbeing of subjects throughout the world. N. A. Christakis, "The Ethical Design of an AIDS Vaccine Trial in Africa," *Hastings Center Report,* 18, 3.June/July (1988) 31–37, p 36.

34. Z. Bankowski. *International Ethical Guidelines for Biomedical Research Involving Human Subjects* (Geneva, Switzerland: Council for International Organizations of Medical Sciences (CIOMS), 1993) 63, p. 6. All participants, their official positions, and their country are listed in an appendix to this document.
35. Z. Bankowski. *International Ethical Guidelines for Biomedical Research Involving Human Subjects* (Geneva, Switzerland: Council for International Organizations of Medical Sciences (CIOMS), 1993) 63, pp 6–7.
36. The principle of confidentiality can be supported, as I have done here, by explaining its value as a protection against social discrimination. The principle may also be defended in its function as a preserver of respect for individual dignity. Consider:

> Respecting confidentiality is a way of respecting the dignity of the patient, of the person who opens himself or herself in body and spirit to the clinician. The pledge of confidentiality, from this perspective, represents a statement, however tacit, that because the patient is vulnerable, a duty exists to treat information provided in the clinical setting with special care, in a manner that will not cause embarrassment or harm. R. Bayer. "Confidentiality and Its Limits." *Ethics and Law in the Study of AIDS.* Eds. H. Fuenzalida-Puelma, A. M. L. Parada and D. S. LaVertu (Washington, DC: Pan American Health Organization, Regional Office of the World Health

Organization, 1992) Scientific Publication No. 530: 145–47, p 145.

Considered from this point of view, as a preserver of respect for persons, how universally applicable is the principle of respect for persons? It is important to note that in considering the applicability of this principle to their own country, none of the CIOMS delegates from developing nations were willing to forgo the application of this principle to their own country. Judith Miller reports thus on the CIOMS consultation discussions:

> Developed in North America with its focus on individualism, how applicable are these values in countries with less individualistic cultural and moral traditions? No participants [in the CIOMS consultations] were willing to discard any of these values for research within their countries, and many acknowledged the need to [re]examine their moral traditions in order to define the most appropriate value framework for ethics review. J. Miller, "Ethical Standards for Human Subject Research in Developing Countries," *IRB, A Review of Human Subjects Research*, 14.3, May–June (1992) 7–8, p 8.

37. Z. Bankowski, ed. *International Ethical Guidelines for Biomedical Research Involving Human Subjects* (Geneva, Switzerland: Council for International Organizations of Medical Sciences (CIOMS), 1993) 63, Guideline 12, p 35. Emphasis mine. Discussion of this Guideline continues in the text (on p 36) and says, in part: "Some jurisdictions require the reporting of, for instance, certain communicable diseases to public health authorities. . . . These and similar limits to the ability to maintain confidentiality should be anticipated and disclosed to prospective subjects."
38. The question as to who should bear the cost of such compensation is controversial. If the private pharmaceutical company which is researching the vaccine is required to bear the cost of compensation (which could be quite substantial), it may be discouraged from even beginning to do research on vaccine development. This has been a problem with development of some vaccines in the past. On the other hand, if a government (or intergovernmental) agency would bear the cost of compensation, it may demand oversight of the research process that would be stifling as only government agencies can be. The World Health Organization may be able to help negotiate such issues of contention between government agencies and private corporations. Global Programme on AIDS. *Potential for WHO-Industry Collaboration on Drug and Vaccine Development for HIV/AIDS* (Geneva: World Health Organization, 1993) 11.
39. Global Programme on AIDS. *Statement from the Consultation on Criteria for International Testing of Candidate HIV Vaccines* (Geneva: World Health Organization, 1989) 13, p 4.
40. D. Hodel and AIDS Action Foundation Working Group. *HIV Preventive Vaccines: Social, Ethical, and Political Considerations* AIDS Action Foundation, Office of AIDS Research, National Institutes of Health, 1994), p 25.

41. Of course, if viruses are not to be considered living things, then they presumably would not be called killed things either. This is, though, commonly used terminology in the vaccine research community.
42. Another type of vaccine under consideration are DNA vaccines, i.e., vaccines that would involve injecting naked DNA into vaccinees. "However, as promising as DNA vaccines may be, there are safety concerns with injecting naked DNA into humans. Theoretically, vaccine DNA might integrate into the host cell chromosome and cause the expression of oncogenes which could lead to tumour formation." W. N. Rida and D. N. Lawrence, "Some Statistical Issues in HIV Vaccine Trials," *Statistics in Medicine,* 13 (1994) 2155–77, p 2157.
43. G. Stine. *Acquired Immune Deficiency Syndrome: Biological, Medical, Social and Legal Issues.* First ed. (Englewood Cliffs, NJ 07632: Prentice Hall, 1993) 462+xxxii, p 214.
44. W. N. Rida and D. N. Lawrence, "Some Statistical Issues in HIV Vaccine Trials," *Statistics in Medicine,* 13 (1994) 2155–77, p 2156. *See also* A. R. Jonsen and J. Stryker, eds. *The Social Impact of AIDS in the United States* (Washington, DC: National Academy Press, 1993) 322+xiv, p 85.
45. A. J. Levine. *Viruses* (New York, NY: Scientific American Library, 1992) 241+xii, p 61.
46. G. Stine. *Acquired Immune Deficiency Syndrome: Biological, Medical, Social and Legal Issues.* First ed. (Englewood Cliffs, NJ 07632: Prentice Hall, 1993) 462+xxxii, p 213.
47. Paul Ewald shows that "unregulated populations increase geometrically rather than arithmetically." P. Ewald. *The Evolution of Infectious Disease* (Oxford University Press, 1994), p 166. He also refers to HIV's special "propensity for evolving resistance and for increasing its rate of replication" (p 167). "HIV therefore seems to make use of two mechanisms to increase net reproduction inside of a host: a high replication rate within cells and rapid generation of genetic variation." (p 154)
48. B. D. Schoub. *AIDS & HIV in Perspective* (New York, NY: Cambridge University Press, 1994) 268+xx, p 185.
49. J. Cohen, "At Conference, Hope for Success Is Further Attenuated," *Science,* 266.18 November (1994) 1154. D. FitzSimons, personal communication, 1994.
50. Dr Ron Desrosier's lab at Harvard's New England Primate Research Center has been working on an attenuated virus vaccine. See J. Cohen, "At Conference, Hope for Success Is Further Attenuated," *Science,* 266.18 November (1994) 1154. See also M. Daniel, et al., "Protective effects of a live attenuated SIV vaccine with a deletion in the nef gene," *Science,* 258 (1992) 1938–41.
51. I think the most important piece of research done on this question is that by Paul Ewald referred to above.
52. P. Ewald, personal communication about virulence, July 15, 1994.
53. "It is . . . inadvisable to give live vaccines to patients being treated with steroids, immunosuppressive drugs or radiotherapy or who have

malignant conditions such as lymphoma and leukaemia; pregnant mothers must also be included here because of the vulnerability of the fetus." I. Roitt. *Essential Immunology*. Seventh ed. (Oxford: Blackwell Scientific Publications, 1991) 356+xii, p 231.

54. B. D. Schoub. *AIDS & HIV in Perspective* (New York, NY: Cambridge University Press, 1994) 268+xx, p 188.

55. B. F. Haynes, "Scientific and Social Issues of Human Immunodeficiency Virus Vaccine Development," *Science*, 260.28 May (1993) 1279–86, p 1282.

   Another form of subunit vaccine is made of peptides which make up the gp120 molecule.

56. D. Hodel and AIDS Action Foundation Working Group. *HIV Preventive Vaccines: Social, Ethical, and Political Considerations* (AIDS Action Foundation, Office of AIDS Research, National Institutes of Health, 1994), p 4.

57. "Unfortunately, however, antibody responses to the immunogen tend to be transient and rapidly fall, even with multiple boosts. A vaccination regimen of four 320-µg doses administered at 0, 1, 6, 12, and 18 months produces antibody responses that are detectable for 6–9 months after immunization by Western blot and EIA assays. However, neutralizing antibodies are seen in only about 30 per cent of vaccines, are of low titer, and are of short duration (3 months) and directed only to the homologous HIV-1." M. J. McElrath and L. Corey. "Current Status of Vaccines for HIV." *Pediatric AIDS: The challenge of HIV infection in infants, children and adolescents.* Eds. P. H. Pizzo and C. M. Wilfert (Baltimore, MD: Williams and Wilkins, 1994) 869–887, p 878.

   See also W. N. Rida and D. N. Lawrence, "Some Statistical Issues in HIV Vaccine Trials," *Statistics in Medicine*, 13 (1994) 2155–77, p 2159.

   As to whether subunit vaccines would protect against only those HIV subtypes for which it was designed, "it is currently not known whether HIV vaccine protective efficacy is HIV subtype dependent." Peter Piot, personal communication, 20 December 1995.

58. D. F. Hoth, et al., "HIV Vaccine Development: A Progress Report," *Annals of Internal Medicine*, 8, 7.15 October (1994) 603–11, p 606. See also J. Crewdson. "AIDS Vaccine Fails Researcher." *Chicago Tribune* Sunday 5 September 1993. 1. Also N. R. Rabinovich, et al., "Vaccine Technologies: View to the Future," *Science*, 265.2 September (1994) 1401–04, p 1403.

   Also: "Live recombinant virus vaccines (vaccines consisting of genetic information from HIV engineered into another virus), such as the vaccinia-HIV recombinant virus currently undergoing Phase I clinical testing [in 1989], pose unique risks associated with the remote possibility of a trial subject transmitting the live recombinant virus from the temporary smallpox-like lesion to another person with whom the trial subject is in close contact." J. P. Porter, M. J. Glass and W. C. Koff, "Ethical Considerations in AIDS Vaccine Testing," *IRB, A Review of Human Subjects Research*, 11 3, May–June (1989) 1–4, p 2.

Also "under field conditions in developing countries, containment [of vaccinia virus and disease] may be more difficult to achieve, so a safer vector is desired." M. J. McElrath and L. Corey. "Current Status of Vaccines for HIV." *Pediatric AIDS: The challenge of HIV infection in infants, children and adolescents.* Eds. P. H. Pizzo and C. M. Wilfert (Baltimore, MD: Williams and Wilkins, 1994) 869–887, p 880.

59. D. A. Henderson and F. Fenner. "Smallpox and Vaccinia." *Vaccines.* Ed. S. A. Plotkin, second ed. (Philadelphia, PA: W.B. Saunders Company, 1994) 13–40, p 19.
60. M. J. McElrath and L. Corey. "Current Status of Vaccines for HIV." *Pediatric AIDS: The challenge of HIV infection in infants, children and adolescents.* Eds. P. H. Pizzo and C. M. Wilfert (Baltimore, MD: Williams and Wilkins, 1994) 869–887, p 880.
61. *Ibid.*
62. *Ibid.*, p 878.
63. E. Blackstone, personal communication about UW's vaccine research studies, July 22, 1994.
64. See Chapter 9 above, on Criteria of Effectiveness.
65. Paul Ewald mentioned 20 years as a possible length of time, or perhaps for the rest of their lives, if we are going to be sure. P. Ewald, personal communication about virulence, July 15, 1994.

> Long-term follow-up is a key component of HIV vaccine efficacy trials. Although blocking infection (sterilizing immunity) must be a primary end point, HIV vaccine efficacy trials should be of sufficient duration to evaluate other end points, including modification of disease progression and long-term safety. . . . Thus several years may be required to assess whether a vaccine modifies or prevents disease. D. Hodel and AIDS Action Foundation Working Group. *HIV Preventive Vaccines: Social, Ethical, and Political Considerations* (AIDS Action Foundation, Office of AIDS Research, National Institutes of Health, 1994), p 12.

The problem of long-term follow-up also plagues those who do efficacy trials for the BCG vaccine, the vaccine that protects against tuberculosis. "This variable, long-term period of dormant infection is one factor that makes BCG vaccine trials so difficult to perform and interpret." J. R. Starke and K. K. Connelly. "Bacille Calmette-Guérin Vaccine." *Vaccines.* Eds. S. A. Plotkin MD and E. A. Mortimer Jr, MD, second ed. (Philadelphia: W. B. Saunders Company, 1994) 439–73, p 441.

66. One vaccine researcher told me that in preliminary studies (probably epidemiological studies) in the Royal Thai Army, researchers were able to achieve only a 60–70 per cent followup rate. That rate seems very low, particularly for people in the army. Military records should make it easier to keep track of individual volunteers in those studies. So a followup rate that low does not bode well for successful monitoring of subjects over a period of years.

Those studies apparently indicated an HIV seroprevalence of around 20 per cent, which would make those army recruits a good group for phase III vaccine trials. G. Eddy, personal communication about HIV vaccine, July 4, 1994.

67. "A control group of subjects (as opposed to a "historical control" group) is essential, because it would be impossible to identify a historical control group that does not differ with regard to risk of HIV infection." D. Hodel and AIDS Action Foundation Working Group. *HIV Preventive Vaccines: Social, Ethical, and Political Considerations* (AIDS Action Foundation, Office of AIDS Research, National Institutes of Health, 1994), p 12.
68. An inert substance used in this way is not properly termed a "placebo," (from the Latin: I shall please). A placebo, in the strict sense, is an inert substance administered in a therapeutic setting which may have a therapeutic effect for a patient due solely to the patient's belief that the substance is curative. This effect is termed the placebo effect. In a looser sense, however, the inert substance administered as a control in a vaccine study may be termed a placebo.
69. D. F. Hoth, et al., "HIV Vaccine Development: A Progress Report," *Annals of Internal Medicine*, 8, 7.15 October (1994) 603–11, p 609.

    Also: "Any possible efficacy of the candidate vaccine could be underestimated if those who believe they have received an effective vaccine increase risk behavior, while those on a placebo diminish sexual risk taking." D. Hodel and AIDS Action Foundation Working Group. *HIV Preventive Vaccines: Social, Ethical, and Political Considerations* (AIDS Action Foundation, Office of AIDS Research, National Institutes of Health, 1994), p 15.

    This could even lead to the paradoxical oddity of vaccinees "experiencing more infections than controls." W. N. Rida and D. N. Lawrence, "Some Statistical Issues in HIV Vaccine Trials," *Statistics in Medicine*, 13 (1994) 2155–77, p 2162.
70. This policy, if chosen, may of course also lead to some problems of test bias, and to possible questions about fair access to candidate vaccine trials.
71. "Others may inadvertently unblind themselves when they donate blood or plasma." W. N. Rida and D. N. Lawrence, "Some Statistical Issues in HIV Vaccine Trials," *Statistics in Medicine*, 13 (1994) 2155–77, p 2162.
72. B. D. Schoub. *AIDS & HIV in Perspective* (New York, NY: Cambridge University Press, 1994) 268+xx, p 186.
73. See Global Programme on AIDS. *Statement from the Consultation on Criteria for International Testing of Candidate HIV Vaccines* (Geneva: World Health Organization, 1989) 13. This document does not explicitly recommend distribution of condoms or clean needles, but it seems to open the door for such a policy. The University of Washington's Vaccine Evaluation Unit does distribute free condoms to volunteers in their phase I/II HIV vaccine trials, though they have not yet seen a need in their population to distribute free needles.

    "The provision of condoms and other barriers to sexual transmission and of the means for sterilizing injection equipment [or, presumably, clean needles] is essential." D. Hodel and AIDS Action

Foundation Working Group. *HIV Preventive Vaccines: Social, Ethical, and Political Considerations* (AIDS Action Foundation, Office of AIDS Research, National Institutes of Health, 1994), p 14.

"It would be unethical to withhold from participants interventions known to be effective in reducing risk behavior." D. Hodel and AIDS Action Foundation Working Group. *HIV Preventive Vaccines: Social, Ethical, and Political Considerations* (AIDS Action Foundation, Office of AIDS Research, National Institutes of Health, 1994), p 13.

74. B. D. Schoub. *AIDS & HIV in Perspective* (New York, NY: Cambridge University Press, 1994) 268+xx, p 189.
75. *Ibid.* p 189–90.

    Dr José Esparza, at WHO's AIDS Vaccine Development Unit, informs me that more recent research indicates that both of these mechanisms are unlikely to occur. Personal communication, March 10, 1995, Geneva.
76. M. Caldwell, "The Long Shot," *Discover*, August (1993) 61–69, pp 68–69. Also B. F. Haynes, "Scientific and Social Issues of Human Immunodeficiency Virus Vaccine Development," *Science*, 260.28 May (1993) 1279–86, p 1283.
77. B. D. Schoub. *AIDS & HIV in Perspective* (New York, NY: Cambridge University Press, 1994) 268+xx, p 190.
78. *Ibid.* Cf also W. C. Koff, "The Next Steps Toward a Global AIDS Vaccine," *Science*, 266.25 November (1994) 1335–37, p 1335.
79. Deborah Blum quotes virologist Nick Lerche, head of the Simian Retrovirus Laboratory at the California primate center, to the same effect: "[E]ven in the so-called benign form, [a whole virus vaccine] might play a little with the human genes. Perhaps, tucked in the body's cells, it might accidentally turn on a genetic switch. By mistake, it could turn on one of the oncogenes, one of the genetic mechanisms that build cancer. When oncogenes flick on, they order abnormal cell growth, turning healthy cells into malignant ones." quoted in D. Blum. *The Monkey Wars* (New York, NY: Oxford University Press, 1994) 306+xii, p 219.
80. G. Bjune and T. W. Gedde-Dahl, "Some problems related to risk-benefit assessments in clinical testing of new vaccines," *IRB*, 15, 1 January–February (1993) 1–5, p 2.
81. *Ibid.*
82. *Ibid.*

    > A single case of such a disease reported during a small-scale trial (phase I or II) should lead to immediate suspension of the trial. Maximal efforts should be made to identify a possible causal relationship with the vaccine. If the chance for a relationship is not negligible, the candidate vaccine should probably be excluded from further clinical testing. pp 2–3.

    No such neuropathies, to my knowledge, have yet been reported in any phase I or II trials of any HIV vaccines.
83. N. A. Christakis, "The Ethical Design of an AIDS Vaccine Trial in Africa," *Hastings Center Report*, 18, 3 June/July (1988) 31–37, p 33.
84. Thalidomide was synthesized by a West German company and

approved for marketing in that country in 1958. Among the twenty countries that approved the over-the-counter sale of thalidomide were Canada, Great Britain, Australia, and Sweden.

While thalidomide was being widely distributed in these countries, physicians noted an alarming increase in the number of children being born with an unusual and extremely rare set of deformities. The most prominent feature was phocomelia, a condition in which the hands are attached to the shoulders and the feet attached to the hips, superficially resembling the flippers of a seal. By 1962, when the link between these birth defects and thalidomide was established, about 8,000 children had been affected.

The harm done to women and their infants by thalidomide was . . . the result of inadequate research (even by contemporary standards), corporate greed, and physicians' uncritical acceptance of promotional claims. . . .

In the United States, a cautious FDA official, Dr Frances Kelsey, delayed marketing approval for thalidomide as an antidote to nausea in early pregnancy. Nevertheless, over 1200 doctors did give their patients thalidomide as an 'investigational' drug. Several thalidomide babies were born in this country as a result, and many more women whose fetuses were affected miscarried. C. Levine, N. N. Dubler and R. J. Levine, "Building a New Consensus: Ethical Principles and Policies for Clinical Research on HIV/AIDS," *IRB*, 13, 1–2 January–April (1991) 1–17, pp 3–4.

See also A. R. Jonsen and J. Stryker, eds. *The Social Impact of AIDS in the United States* (Washington, DC: National Academy Press, 1993) 322+xiv, p 85.

85. Some ethicists have suggested that: "Trial design should also include consideration of a method by which sexual partners of those individuals found to be HIV-infected during the prescreening process can be notified. Any planned notification should be explained early in the informed consent process. Finally, the issue of prescreening the sexual partners of potential vaccine volunteers should be considered in designing protocols for AIDS vaccine trials; thus, the number of persons who are human subjects for purposes of the trial is potentially widened, adding further complexity to informed consent and confidentiality considerations." J. P. Porter, M. J. Glass and W. C. Koff, "Ethical Considerations in AIDS Vaccine Testing," *IRB, A Review of Human Subjects Research*, 11 3, May–June (1989) 1–4, p 2.

   The inclusion of "a method by which sexual partners of those individuals found to be HIV-infected during the prescreening process can be notified" may scare off a certain number of prospective volunteers, and may make it somewhat more difficult to recruit a large enough number of subjects.

86. As an interesting side note, similar scientific problems have faced the development of the BCG vaccine for tuberculosis.

   First, the low incidence of tuberculosis and long incubation period for disease mean that huge study groups must be followed for very long periods of time [10 to 23 years] at great cost. Second, the lack of a serological test for immunity precludes laboratory determination of protection, requiring long-term clinical observation of a large population [one BCG study included 35,000 subjects, another included 88,000 subjects, and another 260,000 subjects]. . . . Also, many of these trials were conducted in developing countries in which resources for diagnosis, vaccination, follow-up, and tracking were inadequate. These challenges as well as the lack of understanding of the immunology involved in protection against tuberculosis make the design and execution of clinical trials extremely difficult. J. R. Starke and K. K. Connelly. "Bacille Calmette-Guérin Vaccine." *Vaccines.* Eds. S. A. Plotkin MD and E. A. Mortimer Jr, MD, second ed. (Philadelphia: W. B. Saunders Company, 1994) 439–73, pp 455–56.

12 Whom Do You Want for Volunteers?

Not just any person will do for phase II and III vaccine trials. What you need is a volunteer who is competent to understand what she or he is getting into, one who has the freedom to give or deny consent, one who is presently HIV negative, and yet one who is still at some fairly high risk for becoming HIV positive. You need a volunteer who is likely to expose himself or herself to the virus. If no subjects ever engaged in risky behaviors, then the vaccine would never be tested against the real virus, and you would never know whether it works or not. The research would be a pointless and expensive waste.

When we are testing candidate vaccines in animal studies, the procedure is simple and clear. We inject the vaccine into the monkey, for example, wait a while for an immune response to develop, then simply "challenge" the immune response by deliberately infecting the monkey with the relevant virus. We then watch to see if the monkey gets sick or not. The test is conceptually straightforward and simple. Now, if we want to find out whether the candidate vaccine will work in human beings, we could theoretically do the same thing: inject subjects with the vaccine, wait for an immune response, then challenge the immune system by deliberately infecting the subjects with wild HIV. This would of course be ethically unacceptable.

Unfortunately, direct challenge vaccine experiments of exactly this sort were actually done using Jewish prisoners at Buchenwald and Natzweiler concentration camps between 1941 and 1945. One experiment, for example, was to test the efficacy of typhus vaccines in human beings. An effective typhus vaccine would have been extremely valuable to the Third Reich, since 1000 soldiers were being lost every day to this disease.[1] The situation was urgent, and a vaccine was desperately needed. For these reasons vaccine experiments involving hundreds of human prisoners were undertaken.

> The general pattern of these typhus experiments was as follows. A group of concentration camp inmates, selected from the healthier ones who had some resistance to disease, were injected with an antityphus vaccine, the efficacy of which was to be tested. Thereafter, all the persons in the group would be infected with typhus. At the same time, other inmates who had not been vaccinated were also infected for purposes of comparison – these unvaccinated victims were called the "control" group.[2]

Similar experiments were done to test the efficacy of spotted fever vaccines.

> In the course of these experiments 75 percent of the selected number of inmates were vaccinated with one of the vaccines . . . and after a period of 3 to 4 weeks, were infected with spotted fever germs. The remaining 25 percent were infected without any previous protection in order to compare the effectiveness of the vaccines.[3]

It is, of course, unethical in the highest degree to deliberately infect human beings with such virulent pathogens. *The Nuremberg Code* was born out of the horror of experiments such as these done by the Nazis.

Perhaps it should not surprise us to learn that similar vaccination experiments were also being done in the US during the war years of the early 1940s, though the experimental vaccines were against influenza rather than against typhus and spotted fever. These experiments, however, did use what we would today classify as vulnerable human subjects, viz., persons in prisons and in mental hospitals, as well as young Army recruits; and these experiments tested the efficacy of the vaccines by the method of direct challenge (i.e., by deliberately infecting subjects) with the pathogen.[4] Influenza is not usually considered to be as virulent a disease with which to be infecting subjects as are typhus and spotted fever, but we should also not forget "The Forgotten Pandemic," viz., the Spanish influenza pandemic of 1918–1919, which did kill approximately 30 million persons around the world in a period of less than 12 months.[5] This is more than the total number of those killed in the fighting of the first World War, and is undoubtedly the reason for the serious US research effort to find a flu vaccine for protection of the military. Influenza is known to have at least the potential to be virulent, and the method of directly challenging experimental subjects with a flu virus is ethically questionable at best. Furthermore, there is no evidence that any of the experimental subjects in the prisons or the mental hospitals were informed about the risks involved in the research, and there is no evidence that those inmates and patients were even asked whether or not they would consent to participate. None of these protocols, therefore, would have been approved by an ethics review committee today.

But we do still have the same research challenges that we had in the 1940s, and we do still need to eventually test our candidate vaccines on human subjects. How, therefore, can such vaccine studies ethically be done? The answer is this: by doing the research on human subjects who will probably be infecting themselves. This is why phase III HIV vaccine trials will need to be done in communities where risk behaviors are common and where the incidence of new HIV infections is high. In fact, the ideal community for doing HIV vaccine trials would be a community in which two conditions obtain: a) the general prevalence of HIV infection is still fairly low, i.e., a large percentage of people in the community are still uninfected, so it will not be difficult to find a large number of sero-negative volunteers. And b) the incidence of new infections is rising steeply, so that your trial population will be more likely to be exposing themselves to the virus.[6] Many Asian nations, some South American nations, and some sub-Saharan African nations, as well as some communities in other parts of the world, fit this profile exactly. (In addition to these two criteria, of course, it will also be important to find communities in which there will be popular and governmental acceptance and support for the research, where research costs will not be high, where circulating HIV subtypes match the candidate vaccines, and where lab facilities, clinical evaluation facilities and facilities for managing the research data are also available.)

Within populations which fit that profile, certain sub-populations may also be targeted for more focused study, including "pre- and postnatal women, commercial sex workers (CSW), injecting drug users (IDU), patients with STDs, homosexual and bisexual men, couples with discordant HIV infection status, university students, workforce employees, and military recruits".[7] Some of these sub-populations will have higher incidence of new infections, and so may be better suited (in some respects) for a vaccine study. On the other hand, some of these sub-populations may have special difficulties that would make them more difficult to follow and monitor in a study.

In any case, for a vaccine trial volunteer group you need subjects who are already, in the regular course of their lives, putting themselves at risk of infection. This is the only way it will be possible to test HIV vaccines on human subjects.

On the other hand you also have a strong moral obligation to "provide clear, thorough and effective counseling to all participants," to strongly urge them to not participate in any risky behaviors, and probably to provide them with condoms and clean needles too. You must intend that your counseling be effective, and you must work to make it truly effective, for all the reasons outlined in Chapter 11, on Real Risks. Yet, if that counseling actually is effective and as a result of the counseling significantly fewer subjects do actually engage in risk behaviors, then a far larger number of subjects will probably be needed to effectively test the candidate vaccine. This will make the trials just that much more expensive, and/or that much lengthier. Or if the counseling is highly effective (as counselors would want it to be), then it could theoretically happen that none (or almost none) of the subjects would engage in risky behaviors. Then the vaccine would never be tested with those subjects.[8]

But you want the vaccine to be tested.

This is a moral dilemma. I call it the dilemma of *counseling with dual intent.* On the one hand you intend your counseling to be effective so as to protect the health and well-being of your subjects. On the other hand, as a researcher you need the vaccine to get tested, and the only way it will get tested is if your subjects go out and expose themselves to the virus. This is the whole point of the research protocol, even if it is never spoken aloud. I cannot imagine any subjects who would not realize what they are being asked to do. It seems that, at some level of consciousness, they will be aware that they are being asked to do two opposite actions: to engage in risk behaviors, and to not engage in risk behaviors.

Responsible researchers should probably have one set of people doing the actual counseling (i.e., trained counselors), another set of people collecting data from subjects about the number of times they have exposed themselves with risky behaviors, and a third set of people monitoring the incoming data to determine whether the vaccine is proving effective or not.[9] This separation of functions (though not yet standard practice in phase I and II trials) may, to some extent, address the problem of counseling with dual intent.[10] But whether even this would eliminate the problem altogether is another question. The entire research protocol, and the entire on-site team, is still clearly giving a mixed message to all volunteers: don't do it, but do it.

NOTES

1. From A. Caplan, "The Doctors' Trial and Analogies to the Holocaust in Contemporary Bioethical Debates," in G. J. Annas and M. A. Grodin, eds. *The Nazi Doctors and the Nuremberg Code: Human Rights in Human Experimentation* (New York, NY: Oxford University Press, 1992) 371+xxii, p 267.
2. From Brig. Gen. Telford Taylor's "Opening Statement of the Prosecution" at the Doctors' Trial, December 9, 1946, in G. J. Annas and M. A. Grodin, eds. *The Nazi Doctors and the Nuremberg Code: Human Rights in Human Experimentation* (New York, NY: Oxford University Press, 1992) 371+xxii, p 81.
3. From the formal indictment read at the final judgment in the Doctors' Trial at Nuremberg, July 1947, in G. J. Annas and M. A. Grodin, eds. *The Nazi Doctors and the Nuremberg Code: Human Rights in Human Experimentation* (New York, NY: Oxford University Press, 1992) 371+xxii, p 99.

   Actually, victims of Nazi biomedical experiments numbered in the hundreds of thousands (p 6).
4. D. J. Rothman. *Strangers at the Bedside: A history of how law and bioethics transformed medical decision making* (Basic Books, Harper Collins, 1991) 303+xii, p 38–39.
5. A. W. Crosby. *America's Forgotten Pandemic: The Influenza of 1918* (New York City, NY: Cambridge University Press, 1989) 337+xiv, p 207.
6. B. D. Schoub. *AIDS & HIV in Perspective* (New York, NY: Cambridge University Press, 1994) 268+xx, p 191.

   Also: "The greater the seroincidence, the fewer subjects will be required and/or the shorter time will be needed to carry out the trial. Populations at high risk (≥ 1% seroincidence) might be considered." D. Hodel and AIDS Action Foundation Working Group. *HIV Preventive Vaccines: Social, Ethical, and Political Considerations* (AIDS Action Foundation, Office of AIDS Research, National Institutes of Health, 1994), p 10.

7. W. L. Heyward, et al., "Preparation for Phase III HIV vaccine efficacy trials: methods for the determination of HIV incidence," *AIDS*, 8, 9 September (1994) 1285–91, p 1286.
8. In addition, if the counseling is highly effective, then the protection results of the candidate vaccine may falsely appear to be very favorable, and thus would seriously bias the results of the study. This could make the candidate vaccine look much more successful than it is in reality. B. D. Schoub. *AIDS & HIV in Perspective* (New York, NY: Cambridge University Press, 1994) 268+xx, p 191.
9. Every trial will already, of course, have an independent Data and Safety Monitoring Board overseeing the progress of the trial. Such a committee monitors the progress of the trial and is able to make recommendations about the continuation, modification, or termination of the trial, if necessary.
10. "Investigators must [in some way] demonstrate that the conflict of interest inherent in the provision of risk-reduction interventions in the course of HIV vaccine efficacy trials is mitigated." D. Hodel and AIDS Action Foundation Working Group. *HIV Preventive Vaccines: Social, Ethical, and Political Considerations* (AIDS Action Foundation, Office of AIDS Research, National Institutes of Health, 1994), p 13.

13 Compensating Volunteers for Injury

Since volunteers will indeed be putting themselves at some degree of risk by their participation in these trials, what responsibilities, if any, will research sponsors have for the treatment and care of injured subjects? Their first responsibility, of course, is to provide medical treatment for any physical problems that may develop in a subject as a result of their participation in the trial. That responsibility is clear and uncontroversial. But what about the emergence of injuries that are not susceptible to medical treatment? How should persons who undergo injuries of this sort be dealt with? And what about the possibility of subjects who may die as a result of their participation in a research protocol? How should their survivors be compensated?

The *International Ethical Guidelines for Biomedical Research Involving Human Subjects* is very clear about the moral obligation of researchers to compensate human subjects for any injuries caused by their participation in an experiment. Guideline 13 of this document, on the "Right of subjects to compensation" reads:

> Research subjects who suffer physical injury as a result of their participation are entitled to such financial or other assistance as would compensate them equitably for any temporary or permanent impairment or disability. In the case of death, their dependents are entitled to material compensation. The right to compensation may not be waived.[1]

This statement of right to compensation seems clear and unambiguous. It is a right that cannot be waived or negotiated away. This principle is important and commendable. On the other hand, in the commentary on this Guideline 13, the document seems to radically limit the actual liability of researchers for providing such compensation. The commentary reads:

> In some societies the right to compensation for accidental injury is not acknowledged. Therefore, when giving their informed consent to participate, research subjects should be told whether there is provision for compensation in case of physical injury, and the circumstances in which they or their dependants would [or would not] receive it.[2]

This enormous limitation of sponsor liability will probably apply to many if not most of the developing nations in which phase III vaccine trials will take place. Countries presently chosen by the Joint United Nations Programme on HIV/AIDS as sites for the first large scale HIV vaccine trials are Brazil, Uganda, and Thailand.[3] I do not know the extent to which these countries presently have laws acknowledging the right to compensation for accidental injury, but even if they do, whether they will still have such laws in five years, or in ten or twenty years, is anybody's guess. In fact in some countries, it is anybody's guess what the overall social and legal structure will be like in five or ten or twenty years when such requests for compensation are likely to be pressed. With the rapidly changing political climate in today's world, it would be difficult to predict what any social structure will be like in twenty years.

If such suits for compensation are pressed against those who sponsored the research (against a pharmaceutical company, for example, or a government agency, or an educational institution), the suits may seek large amounts of compensation and thus may require extensive litigation. It may be an issue whether the legal structure of a developing nation would even be able to support such extensive litigation against a more affluent government or institution. It might also be an issue whether the institution or company that sponsored the research would be able to pay the costs of such compensation, or even whether that sponsor would still be in existence when the suits are pressed.

These considerations might severely limit the likelihood that compensation would ever actually be granted in many cases. Guideline 12, on safeguarding confidentiality (which was discussed above) says that "subjects should be told of the limits to the investigators' ability to safeguard confidentiality." It seems to me that there should be a similar clause in Guideline 13: subjects should be told of the possible limitations on their right to compensation for injury. They should be made aware of the possibility that such compensation might not ever be forthcoming.

Another unsettling limitation on the right to compensation for injury, is that the Guideline focuses exclusively on compensation for *physical* injuries, and says almost nothing about the kinds of real non-physical injuries that can be inflicted by unjust discrimination, for example. All the anti-discrimination laws in developed nations that protect minorities and other disadvantaged persons have been put in place because these societies recognize that there are real injuries other than physical ones. Loss of jobs, loss of housing, loss of income, loss of insurance, loss of medical care, loss of reputation, and so on are just some of the losses recognized by these laws. Why does this Guideline recognize only physical injuries? The answer is probably that the *International Ethical Guidelines for Biomedical Research Involving Human Subjects* is a generic set of guidelines for *all* biomedical research, and not just for research having to do with HIV and AIDS. However, AIDS is a disease that exposes its sufferers to non-physical injuries at least as much as it exposes them to physical injuries. Perhaps this is more true of AIDS than of any other disease in recent history. I believe that ethical guidelines for research involving HIV/AIDS related drugs and vaccines should recognize the likelihood and importance of non-physical injury, and should address that sort of injury at least as thoroughly as it addresses physical injury.[4]

To sum up the matter of compensation for injury: The *International Ethical Guidelines* requires that compensation be promised and made available. Researcher sponsors should recognize and acknowledge the limitations on that "promise," particularly in those developing nations which have changing legal structures and some degree of social instability. They should make those limitations abundantly clear to persons who are considering volunteering for HIV vaccine research. It should be spelled out fully in the process of asking for each volunteer's informed consent.

NOTES

1. Z. Bankowski, ed. *International Ethical Guidelines for Biomedical Research Involving Human Subjects* (Geneva, Switzerland: Council for International Organizations of Medical Sciences (CIOMS), 1993) 63, p 36.
2. *Ibid.* p 37.
3. Rwanda was initially another country on this list, until the "atrocities in Rwanda [in mid-1994] disrupted all normal activities and broke up one of the continent's finest HIV/AIDS research infrastructures." K. M. De Cock MD, MRCP, DTM&H, et al, "The Public Health Implications of AIDS Research in Africa," *JAMA*, 272, 6.10 August (1994) 481–86, p 482.
4. In a section of the *International Ethical Guidelines* not related to compensation for injury, there is mention of the significance of non-physical injury. It reads: "Participation in drug and vaccine trials in the field of HIV infection and AIDS may impose on the research subjects significant associated risks of social discrimination or harm; such risks merit consideration equal to that given to the adverse medical consequences of the drugs and vaccines. Efforts must be made to reduce their likelihood and severity." Z. Bankowski and R. J. Levine, eds. *Ethics and Research on Human Subjects: International Guidelines (Proceedings of the XXVIth CIOMS Conference, Geneva, Switzerland, 5–7 February 1992)* (Geneva, Switzerland: Council for International Organizations of Medical Sciences (CIOMS), 1993) 228+63+x, Guideline 10, p 32.

14 Informed Consent (1)

The principle of informed consent has become almost the cornerstone of medical ethics discussions in the West.[1] Sometimes it seems as if no other principle in medical ethics can hold a candle to the supremacy of this principle. The principle derives its validity from the more basic principle of autonomy, which in turn is based on the even more fundamental principle of respect for persons.[2] In fact the simplest and most profound conclusion of Annas' and Grodin's lengthy 1992 study of the Doctors' Trial at Nuremberg is that "the need to respect the humanity and self-determination of all humans is central to the ethos not only of medicine and human experimentation but of all civilized societies."[3] Even though in recent years ethicists have more and more recognized that there are some limitations on the principle of autonomy, it is still recognized as one of the most important imperatives in all medical ethics decision-making, both in clinical situations and in human subjects research. Many ethicists would argue that, as Annas, Grodin, and Katz put it, "without the informed consent of the competent subject, there really is no defensible justification for using human beings as research subjects."[4] Our focus in these following pages will be on the use of informed consent in biomedical research settings.

In its simplest terms, the principle requires that you tell potential volunteers what the proposed research is about, what you hope to learn by it, what will be expected of them, and what they can expect will happen to them during (and even after) the experiment. Prospective volunteers should also be told what their rights are as participants in the trial, and what their responsibilities are as well. They should probably be given a written "Bill of Rights and Responsibilities" to keep. (I have written, and included in Appendix III, a sample Bill of Rights and Responsibilities for volunteers in HIV vaccine trials.) Prospective volunteers must also be assured that they can quit their participation in the study anytime they wish, without any kind of penalty or cost. Some ethicists have suggested that subjects should also be told what company, institution, or government agency is sponsoring the research, so they can decide whether or not they wish to support that agency's or company's research. Although this is not standard practice right now, it does not seem like an unreasonable recommendation.

At least as important as the content of what they must be told, subjects must also be able to competently deliberate and freely choose, "without the intervention of any element of force, fraud, deceit, duress, overreaching, or other ulterior form of constraint or coercion."[5]

In its simplest terms, this is what the principle requires. In practice, things are rather more complex. And when investigators are doing research in developing nations, yet another layer of complexity is added to an already troublesome tangle of issues.

Several functions are intended to be served by application of this principle. The principle is partly intended to promote self-reflection in the biomedical research community and to promote self-scrutiny and rational decision-making among investigators. But the principle's primary function is to promote the autonomy of individuals and to insure the protection of vulnerable subjects.

Applying this principle to each individual volunteer may be much more difficult in developing nations, where levels of literacy are much lower than in developed nations, where beliefs about the nature and causation of disease may be different from those held by the researchers, and where the notion and value of personal identity and individuality may be strikingly different than that held in Western nations. Because of these factors the principle of informed consent, which has been one of the cornerstones of biomedical ethics since its origins in *The Nuremberg Code,* will be problematic in developing nations.

And yet the ethical guidelines are very clear: ethical standards governing human subjects research must be no less stringent in developing nations than they are in developed nations. *International Ethical Guidelines* 15 is quite explicit: when a sponsoring agency submits its research proposal to ethical review in the country of origin (as it is required to do), the "ethical standards applied [to research in developing nations] should be no less exacting than they would be in the case of research carried out in that country [of origin]."[6]

This single sentence alone underlines one of the key problems faced by research sponsors: conditions in some underdeveloped communities may be significantly different than in developed communities, yet the ethical standards must be applied just as stringently as they are anywhere. This is good ethics, but it presents researchers with some almost insurmountable problems. There must be utmost regard for individual autonomy in decision making. *Every single subject* must be *fully* informed and must give free consent. "The investigator is required to ensure that *each prospective subject* is clearly told *everything* that would be conveyed if the study were to be conducted in a developed community."[7]

"Everything?" the intelligent reader might ask. "Everything," emphasizes the *Guidelines.* That will include a variety of kinds of information, including "the aims and methods of the research; the expected duration of the subject's participation; . . . any foreseeable risks or discomfort to the subject; . . . the extent to which confidentiality of records in which the subject is identified will be maintained; . . . whether the subject or the subject's family or dependants will be compensated for disability or death,"[8] and all the possible harms and hazards that may be attendant on participating in the research.

In the case of HIV vaccine research specifically, this principle requires informing prospective subjects about what a vaccine is and what an immune system is, as well as about

> the concepts of randomization, blinding [and double-blinding], placebos, informed consent, and risk/benefit, concepts which [may not be] easily understood in the cultural context of many developing countries.[9]

Ethical guidelines require that prospective research subjects be fully informed of all these aims, purposes, methodologies, and hazards associated with their participation in research protocols for which they are considering volunteering.

NOTES

1. Already by 1983 there had been over 4000 journal articles published on this single subject alone R. J. Levine. *Ethics and Regulation of Clinical Research,* second ed. (New Haven, CT: Yale University Press, 1986, 1988) 452+xx, p x.
2. *See* Chapter 10 above, on Ethical Principles.
3. G. J. Annas and M. A. Grodin, eds. *The Nazi Doctors and the Nuremberg Code: Human Rights in Human Experimentation* (New York, NY: Oxford University Press, 1992) 371+xxii, p 7.
4. *Ibid.*, p 313.
5. *The Nuremberg Code, see* Appendix II.
6. Z. Bankowski, ed. *International Ethical Guidelines for Biomedical Research Involving Human Subjects* (Geneva, Switzerland: Council for International Organizations of Medical Sciences (CIOMS), 1993) 63, p 43.
7. *Ibid.*, p 27 (emphasis mine).
8. *Ibid.*, Guideline 2, p 14.
9. W. L. Heyward, et al., "Preparation for Phase III HIV vaccine efficacy trials: methods for the determination of HIV incidence," *AIDS*, 8, 9 September (1994) 1285–91, p 1289.

   Such simple concepts may not even be understood in developed nations. Stine tells the following story:

   "A heterosexual client at an HIV/AIDS clinic and the counselor became involved in a discussion of the client's sexual behavior. The counselor was concerned and somewhat confused when the client insisted that anal intercourse was not a risky sexual behavior. The counselor responded with a set of facts that led to the inescapable conclusion that anal intercourse was a very risky sexual behavior. The client said 'Gee, you wouldn't think that having sex once a year would place you at high risk for HIV infection.' It was immediately obvious to the counselor that the client's lack of understanding resulted from confusing the words annual and anal." G. Stine. *Acquired Immune Deficiency Syndrome: Biological, Medical, Social and Legal Issues.* First ed. (Englewood Cliffs, NJ 07632: Prentice Hall, 1993) 462+xxxii, p 322.

15 Assessing Comprehension

Nor is it enough to simply provide information to prospective subjects. In addition to that, there must also be a determined and good faith effort on the part of researchers to ascertain whether or not the prospective subject has heard and adequately *understood* what you have told him or her.[1] The basic underlying intent of the requirement for informed consent, after all, is for researchers to insure that prospective subjects understand the purposes, procedures, risks, etc. of the research, i.e., that they have in their minds the full measure of information necessary for making an informed and free choice. Simply reading information, facts or data to a prospective subject does not satisfy the intent of the principle of informed consent, particularly when "the potential for misunderstanding is considerable," as it will be with AIDS vaccine trials.[2] The intent of the principle is to insure that each prospective subject fully understands what they might be getting themselves into, so they can make a good decision based on adequate and true information.

If this is true, then it is imperative that researchers make a serious, good faith effort to assess the degree to which subjects have actually heard and comprehended the information that has been conveyed to them. An important question, therefore, is: after providing all the requisite information to prospective subjects, just how might such an assessment of the level of their understanding be adequately accomplished?

Fortunately, this is not a new problem. Teachers and professors for centuries have faced this problem almost daily. Teachers and professors know well that simply giving a lecture, or providing lecture notes, or assigning a good text is not by itself sufficient to insure that the student has actually comprehended the material. I am a professor at a community college and I teach adults, most of whom have come back to school because they are highly motivated to learn and earn a college degree. And yet, in spite of all their good will and strong motivation, students often simply do not "get" the information that professors try to provide them. The information does not register, for any number of reasons. Perhaps the student was distracted that day, or was not feeling well, or was busy worrying about some other issue in his or her life, or perhaps simply did not understand the importance of what they had been told. So they did not learn it. Part of the professor's task, in addition to teaching the necessary material, is to be continually assessing the degree to which students are understanding it.

The reasons for doing this assessment of their understanding are twofold: a) so that you can see what they have understood so far, in order to do a better job of teaching the material still to come (the so-called "formative" evaluation), and b) to make a final assessment of whether they registered enough of the material for you to certify that they now understand it (the so-called "summative" evaluation).

At least the second purpose, the summative one, if not the first, will be important for researchers. They will have to be able to determine whether prospective subjects understood enough of the material they were told so that they could now make an informed decision about whether to participate in the trials or not.

How might researchers make such an assessment of understanding? Is it enough to, at the end of a presentation, simply ask "Did you understand all that?" Every teacher knows that that is hardly a satisfactory assessment technique. Is it enough to look into a student's eyes, after they have been given information, and tell by the understanding look in their eyes that they have comprehended the material? That, of course, is not adequate either. The most common manner of dealing with the problem of assessment is to require that students take some manner of test.

Methods of testing, of course, are almost limitless in their variety. They range from true/false and multiple choice tests (which actually are very poor indicators of student comprehension), through fill-in-the-blank tests (which are slightly better indicators of understanding), to short essay tests, longer essay tests, and oral response tests. Whatever method of testing is ultimately determined best for assessing the understanding of prospective subjects after they have been given information about their participation in a vaccine trial, it is at least clear that some method of assessing understanding will be necessary. Ethics Review Committees (ERCs) will probably require that researchers have designed a clear method of assessing understanding, and have explained the manner in which they will administer it.[3]

Additional questions, however, will still need to be dealt with: it will need to be determined what percentage of understood information is acceptable for prospective subjects; 70 per cent is often a good enough score to pass tests in a college course. ERCs will have to decide whether it is acceptable if prospective volunteers understand only 70 per cent of the information given to them. Will it be acceptable, for example, if they do not understand how a condom is used, or what the value is in using it, but they do understand most of the rest of the material? Will it be acceptable if they do not understand the risks involved in the probable social discrimination which could result from their participation in the trial, but they do understand most of the rest of the material? Will it be acceptable if they do not understand that they might receive a placebo, or that there may be some physical risks involved, or that they will need to give blood periodically, or that they will probably seroconvert to HIVAb+ and what that means, or that the candidate vaccine is not a proven vaccine at all, etc.? In other words, are there any *essential* pieces of information that it will be imperative for them to understand, such that without that understanding they could not be allowed to consent to participate in the trial? That is, is any of the information in the informed consent procedure essential information, information they must have in order to participate? If any of the information is essential, then they will need to understand all of that essential information. If they are tested on the essentials, they will need to show that they have understood 100 per cent of that essential information. Understanding 80 per cent of it, or even 90 per cent of it, will not be acceptable.

Earning 100 per cent on any test is rather a difficult chore, as most of us know by humbling experience. Will a test, then, contain some items that test for understanding of essential material, and some items that test for understanding of material that is not essential? Should it be absolutely required to understand some of the items on the test, but on other items it would be sufficient to understand only 70 per cent of them? Or might there be two separate tests administered, one of which tests for essential information, and the other of which tests for merely important information? Would it then be necessary to score 100 per cent on the one test, and 70 per cent on the other one?

Or perhaps it will be argued that testing of this sort is too heavy a burden to place on prospective volunteers. Perhaps, it may be said, such testing requirements will discourage many potential subjects from even offering to participate in a trial. Might a requirement of this sort, in fact, discourage so many prospective volunteers that it would make procurement of enough volunteers an even more daunting task than it is already. When we realize how difficult it is going to be to find cohorts of several thousand (or tens of thousands of) volunteers for phase III trials, might it be that these testing requirements will simply place one more high hurdle in the way of well-intentioned researchers?

In addition, might testing of this sort end up actually biasing (i.e., reducing the randomness of) the cohort of test volunteers by selecting for those volunteers who find it easier to learn information and take tests? This could run the risk of introducing a socioeconomic bias into the selection of cohorts if there turns out to be any correlation between socioeconomic grouping and familiarity with test-taking, or ease of test-taking.

These are difficult issues. And, much as we might be tempted to overlook them, these issues simply cannot be ignored or dismissed. The principle of informed consent is absolutely essential to all research involving human subjects, to such an extent that without fully informed consent, no research with human subjects would probably be justifiable at all. But that principle requires that prospective subjects actually comprehend the information that has been given to them. If the principle does require that subjects understand the information before they are asked for their consent, then researchers will need to design methods of accurately assessing whether or not prospective subjects have understood the information given to them. Only then is it likely that ERCs will allow researchers to ask for subjects' consent.

These would seem to be heavy demands to place on researchers, if looked at from the researchers' point of view. Those who hold the Antithesis position insist, however, that requirements such as these are necessary if we are to adequately demonstrate respect for the autonomy of the volunteers participating in these trials. In demonstrating this respect, they say, there must be no exceptions.

NOTES

1. "When the trials actually get underway, it will be necessary to study the effectiveness of the whole informed consent process, including studies of the various means for assessing volunteers' comprehension of the material given to them." D. Hodel and AIDS Action Foundation Working Group. *HIV Preventive Vaccines: Social, Ethical, and Political Considerations* (AIDS Action Foundation, Office of AIDS Research, National Institutes of Health, 1994), p 26.
2. "Comprehending the difference between a vaccine-induced positive antibody test, for example, and a virus-induced positive antibody test, and the social consequences of each, will be important information, but may require a good bit of explaining before subjects fully understand it." D. Hodel and AIDS Action Foundation Working Group. *HIV Preventive Vaccines: Social, Ethical, and Political Considerations* (AIDS Action Foundation, Office of AIDS Research, National Institutes of Health, 1994), p 2.
3. One vaccine research laboratory was good enough to send me a copy of the rather minimalist true/false test which they use to assess comprehension in their HIV vaccine trial subjects. I have included a copy of this test (with identifiers stripped off) as Appendix IV in this book. Readers will need to decide for themselves whether they think this test is an adequate assessment of all the necessary information trial subjects should have before they can give any valid consent to participate in the trial.

16 Informed Consent (2)

Even the urgency of our global situation, even the fact that we are in the midst of a serious pandemic in which the number of new infections every hour is accelerating, even these urgencies, says the Antithesis position, should not allow ethical guidelines, especially those relating to informed consent, to be relaxed. The Nazi doctors certainly felt that the urgent demands of a major war effort justified taking ethical shortcuts in their medical experiments with human beings, but the condemnations of the Nuremberg trials have made that kind of thinking unacceptable ever since. The Antithesis position insists that even today's urgencies must not be used as an excuse for taking ethical shortcuts in human subjects research. "The life-threatening and infectious nature of HIV/AIDS does not justify any suspension of the rights of research subjects to informed consent."[1]

The question one is then left with is: will it actually be possible to *fully* inform *all* prospective subjects? The answer to this question will be difficult. Ethics Review Committees will need to decide how best to apply the principle of informed consent in developing nations. That the principle of requiring informed consent from each individual research subject does and should apply, virtually all ethicists (including those from developing nations) do seem to believe. Given this reality, we must now face questions about how best to implement the principle in cultures where it did not originate.

The principle of informed consent is articulated in Guideline 1 of *The International Ethical Guidelines for Biomedical Research Involving Human Subjects.*

> For all biomedical research involving human subjects, the investigator must obtain the informed consent of the prospective subject or, in the case of an individual who is not capable of giving informed consent, the proxy consent of a properly authorized representative.[2]

The astute reader will already have noticed the caveat, "in the case of the individual who is not capable of giving informed consent." In medical ethics discussions in the past five decades, this phrase has been primarily applied to individual clinical patients who are a) too young to give legal consent, or b) are comatose (or virtually comatose), or c) are judged to be in some way *non compos mentis*, perhaps due to mental retardation, advanced age or some mentally incapacitating disease process (either physical or psychological). The thinking has been that for an individual who is not "competent" to give consent, the "proxy consent"[3] of someone who represents the patient, and who is authorized to express the wishes of the patient, will be accepted in his or her stead. As far as I know, the principle of proxy consent has been applied almost exclusively in clinical situations.

The application of the proxy consent principle to subjects in biomedical research has been much less common. Where it has been applied to research, it has been in situations that are a mix of therapy and research where, for example, a non-competent patient could be given access to an *experimental* drug or procedure which also has potential therapeutic value. The purposes to be served in using the experimental drug or procedure are twofold: there is both a therapeutic purpose for the potential benefit of that individual patient, and there is a research related purpose in which we want to know more about that drug or procedure. In dual purpose situations of this nature, proxy consent has been used. Very rarely have any pure research situations resorted to the proxy consent principle.

The "Commentary on Guideline 1" in *The International Ethical Guidelines* contains a paragraph which may be applicable to this question of proxy consent. It deserves to be quoted at length:

> When the research design involves no more than *minimal* risk – that is, risk that is no more likely and not greater than that attached to routine medical or psychological examination – and it is *not practicable to obtain informed consent from each subject* (for example, where the research involves only excerpting data from subjects' records) the ethical review committee may waive some or all of the elements of informed consent. Investigators should never

initiate research involving human subjects without obtaining *each subject's* informed consent, *unless they have received explicit approval* to do so from an ethical review committee.[4]

This commentary emphasizes the importance, in all human subjects research, of obtaining *each individual subject's* informed consent. Two exceptions are allowed. (I have flagged both with italics.) The first exception applies only when two conditions are both present: a) when there is minimal risk, and b) when it is not practicable to obtain informed consent from each subject. In phase III HIV vaccine trials in developing nations, the second condition may well apply, i.e., it may be very difficult to obtain informed consent from each subject. The first condition, however, that the experiment involve only minimal risk clearly does not apply, as we have seen above in Chapter 11, on Real Risks.

Might the other exception, viz., receiving explicit approval from an ethics review committee to dispense with "obtaining each subject's informed consent" apply to such trials? That is unknown right now, but if it did happen, it would require:

1 that research sponsors provide to the Ethics Review Committee a list of solid reasons why it would be *ethically* acceptable to dispense with informed consent from each subject; and
2 that sponsors also suggest alternate procedures which would provide support for the autonomy of individual subjects and would protect vulnerable subjects, since these are two of the main goals of the informed consent principle.

Having heard these reasons and alternate procedures, the Ethics Review Committee would then deliberate, make its decision, and the decision, presumably, would be final.

In any case, and by whatever method research sponsors choose to obtain the informed consent of subjects, that such consent will be necessary in HIV vaccine trials is absolutely clear. Informed consent is required by virtually all codes of medical conduct written and promulgated, both nationally and internationally, since Nuremberg. The requirement is also part of international law and is even included in the United Nations International Covenant on Civil and Political Rights, promulgated in 1966 and adopted by the UN General Assembly in 1974. Specifically, article 7 of the covenant reads:

> No one shall be subjected to torture or to cruel, inhuman or degrading treatment or punishment. In particular, no one shall be subjected without his free consent to medical or scientific experimentation.[5]

It is the ERC's responsibility to ensure that the requirement for getting individual informed consent from each subject is adequately met by the research sponsors.

It is probably not likely that the review committee would take measures to oversee the actual ongoing research to insure that ethical standards were being followed, but the committee will probably require annual review of the protocols to determine compliance with ERC requirements. Then if reasons for suspicion developed, the committee would certainly be able to withdraw its approval of the protocol and could in the future require stringent, on-site oversight procedures to insure compliance.

There have actually already been allegations of serious ethical misconduct in the performance of early HIV vaccine trials. There have been accusations of intentionally initiating vaccine trials in developing nations where there were as yet no provisions for ethical review of research, in hopes of having less strict oversight over research. There have been allegations of trying untested HIV vaccines on small children who are too young to know what is happening to them. There have been charges of withholding data about the deaths of vaccinated subjects from published reports of vaccine experiments in order to make the results look better than they actually were. There have been charges of surreptitious alteration of government patent documents to cover up possible misconduct.[6] These are all only allegations, of course, and may well prove to have no validity at all. After all, anyone can make any allegations. But if such allegations were found to have some merit, an ERC would almost certainly withdraw approval from the involved protocols, and this would doubtless have the effect of terminating all funding for the project. The research would then be out of business until it could be shown that the protocol was back in formal compliance with all ethical requirements.

NOTES

1. Z. Bankowski, ed. *International Ethical Guidelines for Biomedical Research Involving Human Subjects* (Geneva, Switzerland: Council for International Organizations of Medical Sciences (CIOMS), 1993) 63, p 32.
2. *Ibid.*, p 13.
3. *See* Chapter 19 on Proxy Consent?
4. Z. Bankowski, ed. *International Ethical Guidelines for Biomedical Research Involving Human Subjects* (Geneva, Switzerland: Council for International Organizations of Medical Sciences (CIOMS), 1993) 63, pp 13–14 (my emphasis).
5. G. J. Annas and M. A. Grodin, eds. *The Nazi Doctors and the Nuremberg Code: Human Rights in Human Experimentation* (New York, NY: Oxford University Press, 1992) 371+xxii, p 311.
6. J. Crewdson. "AIDS Vaccine Fails Researcher." *Chicago Tribune* Sunday 5 September 1993, 1.

17 Ethics Review Committees

What exactly are Ethics Review Committees? They are usually associated with an institution, such as a university, a company, or a government agency within a nation. In addition, some are independent, private, for-profit companies. These committees go by different names in different countries. In the US such committees are called Human Subjects boards, or (more officially) Institutional Review Boards (IRBs). They were given this official designation by the US Congress in 1974.[1] In Canada they are called Research Ethics Boards (REBs), and in the UK they are usually referred to as Ethical Committees (ECs).[2] I have simply referred to them as Ethics Review Committees (ERCs) since this seems the most descriptive designation for what these committees actually do. There are not presently any international Ethics Review Committees (though WHO has recently begun to give some consideration to the idea of an international ERC). But as of now, all ERCs are either national in scope, or local, i.e., associated with an institution or an agency within a nation. What this means is that ethics policy normally is determined within individual countries. In fact, even if there is an international Ethics Review Committee in existence when the first candidate vaccines are ready for phase III trials (i.e., an ERC with international "authority" to recommend policy), CIOMS *Guidelines* still require that the research protocol pass ERC review both in the country of origin, and in the country or countries where the trials will take place.[3] Even if there are internationally focused ERCs, ethical review will still need to be done in the country hosting the trial.

As a brief aside, it will be worth mentioning that researchers in the US will probably not experience any conflicting or contradictory requirements in the two sets of guidelines that they will be expected to satisfy in an ethical review for protocols to be done in developing nations. One set of guidelines they will be expected to satisfy, of course, is the CIOMS *International Ethical Guidelines for Biomedical Research Involving Human Subjects* which we have been examining in this book, and the other is the US Department of Health and Human Services *Regulations for the Protection of Human Subjects*, embodied in the Code of Federal Regulations as 45 CFR 46.[4] These latter regulations are the formal guidelines already being used by today's ERCs in the US when they are performing ethical review of biomedical protocols. A quick search for significant conflicts or contradictions between these two sets of guidelines will reveal that US researchers will probably not have to deal with any significant differences in either spirit or intent between the two sets of guidelines.

There are differences, of course, but these stem primarily from the fact that the two sets of guidelines are written in two different genres of literature. One, the HHS Regulations, is part of a legal code, and was framed, constructed, and worded primarily by legislators and attorneys. It is written in language that is closer to "legalese" than it is to ordinary discourse. While it is true that the regulations in 45 CFR 46 were partially inspired by the deliberations and recommendations of The National Commission for the Protection of Human Subjects (a deliberative and philosophical, rather than a legalistic body),[5] still the language is primarily the language of the lawmaker. Sentences such as "Compliance with these regulations will in no way render inapplicable pertinent federal, state, or local laws or regulations," exemplify the language of this set of regulations.

The CIOMS *Guidelines*, on the other hand, are not (as we have seen) written by legislators and do not have the ring of legislative statute-making. They have the ring, instead, of the ethical code, the moral regulation, the conscientious demand of simple good sense. They were, after all, arrived at by long rational deliberation of good people trying to articulate what they believed to be most fair and just. The CIOMS *Guidelines* are, therefore, an entirely different genre of literature.

Both sets of guidelines, moreover, are equally clear about the importance of protecting each individual research subject, about the importance of taking special care to protect vulnerable subjects, such as children, prisoners,[6] the elderly, the mentally incompetent, and so on, and about the importance of the requirements for informed consent. Both documents emphasize the importance of a fair balance between risks and benefits, compensation in the event of research-related injuries, and so on. Researchers in the US, who are designing trials that will be done both in the US (perhaps) and in developing nations, and who will probably need to satisfy both sets of guidelines in order for their research to be approved, should not experience any conflicts between these two sets of guidelines.

In any case, the reason for the requirement that ethical review be done both in the country of origin (where the candidate vaccine was developed and manufactured) and in the host country (where the trials will take place) is that the power of Ethics Review Committees to approve or disapprove research protocols can be very influential in insuring that ethical principles are maintained. In US history, for example, a number of studies using human subjects were able to be done only because there were no ERCs in existence at the time they were undertaken. Examples are numerous. Besides the vaccine trials mentioned above, there was also the infamous Willowbrook, New York hepatitis study which undertook to observe the effects of deliberately infecting institutionalized retarded children with hepatitis. The Tuskegee syphilis study observed the effects of untreated syphilis on black males in Macon County, Alabama, even after an effective treatment for syphilis was available, and without ever obtaining proper informed consent from any of the subjects. There have also been over 1400 US government-backed human radiation experiments, conducted between 1944 and 1975, involving the exposure of approximately 23,000 human beings to nuclear radiation.[7] There have also been studies (in the 1960s) observing the effects of LSD on unsuspecting army recruits, and numerous other less well known experiments that were also able to be done only because there were no ERCs in existence. None of these experiments would come close to passing ethical review in any of today's ERCs.

Of course, the mere existence of ERCs does not guarantee that there will be no ethically questionable research with human subjects. A recent news story suggests that the US Pentagon engaged in experimental use of vaccines during the Persian Gulf War in 1990 and 1991, without obtaining informed consent from army recruits and reservists. Some troops, apparently, were even "threatened with punishment if they did not obey orders to take the chemicals. . . . Many Gulf War veterans also were ordered to tell no one about their [experimental] vaccinations."[8] ERCs were not able to prevent these experimental studies because the studies were never required to undergo ethical review. These studies may not have passed ethical review, and perhaps would not even have passed scientific review, at the time they were instigated. The FDA simply made an exception and allowed the vaccines to be used without any ethical review, probably because the country was at war. (If nothing else, these studies should make us more than a little suspicious of the ability to obtain free and uncoerced consent from military recruits in any country, particularly in countries without strong civil rights traditions.)

Nonetheless, even though the existence of ERCs does not guarantee that all experiments with human subjects will be ethical, the existence of these committees does at least increase the likelihood that human subjects in biomedical research protocols will be protected.

NOTES

1. R. J. Levine. *Ethics and Regulation of Clinical Research.* Second ed. (New Haven, CT: Yale University Press, 1986, 1988) 452+xx, p 328.
2. J. Miller, "Ethical Standards for Human Subject Research in Developing Countries," *IRB, A Review of Human Subjects Research,* 14.3, May–June (1992) 7–8, p 8.
3. Z. Bankowski, ed. *International Ethical Guidelines for Biomedical Research Involving Human Subjects.* (Geneva, Switzerland: Council for International Organizations of Medical Sciences (CIOMS), 1993) 63, Guideline 15, p 43.
4. Enacted May 30, 1974. R. J. Levine. *Ethics and Regulation of Clinical Research.* Second ed. (New Haven, CT: Yale University Press, 1986, 1988) 452+xx, p xi.
5. *Ibid.*, pp xi–xiii.

6. One wonders why there is no recognition in either document that military recruits are in some ways also vulnerable subjects, whose ability to give free consent may also be somewhat compromised.
7. W. P. &. S. T. Staff. "Radiation tests involved at least 23,000." *Seattle Times* 22 October 1994, A1.
8. C. Burrell for the Associated Press. "Report: 'Reckless' use of Gulf War drugs." *Seattle Times* 8 December 1994, A3.

18 Protecting Individual Subjects

Herein lies the importance of Ethics Review Committees for human subjects research.

18.1 INDIVIDUAL VOLUNTEERS ARE PROTECTED

The primary function of the ERC is to oversee and insure the protection of the individual human beings who will be volunteering for this particular research protocol.

> [A]ccording to the National Commission [for the Protection of Human Subjects of Biomedical and Behavioral Research], the primary purpose of the IRB is to assist the investigator in safeguarding the rights and welfare of human research subjects.[1]

The primary charge of these committees to insure the protection of human subjects must be underscored. The US Department of Health and Human Services established its ethics policy (in 1983) for ethical review of "all research involving human subjects conducted by the Department of Health and Human Services or funded in whole or in part by [the Department, as well as all] research conducted or funded [by HHS] outside the United States."[2] This policy is now federal law,[3] and is titled "Basic HHS Policy for Protection of Human Research Subjects." The whole focus of this law is on the responsibility of the IRB "for protecting the rights and welfare of human subjects of research."[4] The clear thrust of *The Nuremberg Code* also, as well as the thrust of the CIOMS *Guidelines* is in their mandate to safeguard the rights and welfare of subjects participating in medical research. As Robert Levine, one of the principal authors of the CIOMS *Guidelines* says in his earlier landmark publication, *Ethics and Regulation of Clinical Research,* "The primary purpose of the IRB is essentially as stated by the Surgeon

General in 1966: to safeguard the rights and welfare of human research subjects."[5]

I underscore this primary charge of the ERCs at some length because of a fundamental problem that can easily occur in our thinking about ethical review of human subjects research. The problem I refer to is the mistake of weighing the risks borne by *individual* subjects against potential benefits that might accrue to *society at large.* In the concentration camps, for example, individual research subjects from the camps were the ones enduring the burdens and harms of the research, and the benefits of the research were supposed to accrue (at least in the best case) to society at large. We might, for example, imagine one of the Nazi doctors, perhaps one with a small bit of conscience, thinking "Yes, it is too bad that these individual prisoners must suffer in our experiments, but their suffering will at least work for the greater good of society, and for the good of many thousands of human beings to come."

One of the Nazi doctors tried at Nuremberg did, in fact, express exactly these rationalizations. Dr Gerhard Rose, head of the Koch Institute of Tropical Medicine in Berlin during the war, said that

> while he initially opposed performing lethal experiments on camp inmates, he came to believe that it made no sense not to involve 100 or 200 people in research, even lethal research, in pursuit of a vaccine for typhus when the Reich was losing 1000 men a day to this disease on the Eastern front. What, he asked, were the deaths of 100 men compared to the possible benefit of developing a prophylactic vaccine capable of saving tens of thousands?[6]

Philosophers term this approach to moral decision making – i.e., the attempt to make moral judgments based on a quantification of the costs and benefits of human acts – the utilitarian approach. This approach originated with British thinkers Jeremy Bentham (1748–1832) and John Stuart Mill (1806–1873), and has always appealed to those who would like to find a way to quantify human happiness and suffering as a way of simplifying, or clarifying, moral decision-making.

Because the Nuremberg Tribunals found this particular application of a utilitarian justification of human suffering so odious, at least in the way it was being applied to medical experiments in the camps, the ethical principles of *The Nuremberg Code* were formulated to require researchers to protect the health and well-being of every single individual human subject in their experiments. The philosophy behind the Doctors' Trials at Nuremberg, whether articulated fully or not, was that human beings have worth in themselves, and are not merely to be used as a means for the benefit of others, even if that benefit is very great. It was in fact the German philosopher Immanuel Kant (1724–1804) who is most noted for enunciating this principle late in the 18th century: "So act as to treat humanity, whether in thine own person or in that of any other, in every case as an end withal, never as a means only."[7]

For these reasons, when ERCs review proposed human subjects protocols, they look for a balance of harms and benefits *for these individual subjects.* What potential benefits might accrue to these subjects, and what potential harms? They do not ask what potential harms might come to these individual subjects and what potential benefits might come to society at large. Dr Claude Bernard, one of the classical formulators of medical research ethics in the 19th century, summarizes this point very succinctly:

> The principle of medical and surgical morality [he wrote in 1865] consists in never performing on man an experiment which might be harmful to him to any extent, even though the result might be highly advantageous to science, i.e., to the health of others.[8]

Even today, an AIDS Action Foundation working group on the design of HIV vaccine trials states very clearly: "The hope for social benefit must never be used to justify excessive risk to individual subjects."[9]

I emphasize this point at length because in HIV vaccine research there may be a temptation to ask the harm/benefit question in just these terms, viz., in terms of harms risked by individual subjects balanced against benefits to society at large. One recent author does in fact (though I think not consciously) weigh the risks and benefits of HIV vaccine research in exactly these terms (i.e., risks to the individual subjects weighed against potential benefits to society).[10] He is not alone, however. "The need for a vaccine is so urgent," I have heard one AIDS activist intone, "that subjects in vaccine trials may just have to take greater than normal risks; we simply cannot wait for the ethicists to realize how serious the need is!"

Some may argue, of course, that it is

> difficult to see how the interests of the subject conflict with the interests of the society except, of course, if the society is not his own. That is, the interest of the subject and of society are necessarily congruent. Problems arise only if the values and expectations of a society of which the individual is not a member are imposed upon him.[11]

Christakis is here referring to a perspective that an African may have. I suspect that it is also a perspective that an ancient Greek may have had about his polis, and probably a perspective that is shared today by some persons in closely knit communities. Grady also argues that the benefits accruing to a community should be weighed into the equation for determining the ethical value of a clinical trial, particularly the value of a vaccine trial.[12] Vaccines, after all, do benefit the community at least as much as they benefit individuals.

Nevertheless, it seems to me that this consideration does not diminish the critical importance of the requirement to fully inform each individual subject, to fully respect each subject's individual autonomy, and to fully respect each subject's right to make a free choice about whether to volunteer for a trial or not. The WHO/CIOMS *Guidelines* are clear in their requirement to protect the autonomy of each individual subject, no matter how serious the community need for a vaccine may be.

And I think most of us do realize how serious the need is. If you have considered the information in the first chapters of this book on the present state and expected future course of the epidemic, you too realize how urgent the need is. Ethics Review Committees will also be aware of the epidemic's urgency, and they will be pursuing their deliberations and making their decisions in the thick of such urgency. Yet their primary responsibility continues to be to protect the health and the overall physical, social and psychological well-being of the individual human subjects in these studies.

Some cynical critics, of course, do not see ERCs as serving any real ethical purpose at all, and certainly do not see them as a force for protecting the research volunteers. These cynical critics see ERCs simply as committees for protecting the legal and economic interests of the companies and agencies to which they are attached, not as committees for protecting the interests of research subjects. These critics believe that pharmaceutical companies, government agencies, universities and other private and public institutions have ERCs only for the purpose of minimizing their legal and economic risks due to research. Unfortunately, this cynical view may be true more often than we would wish (some think it is more true of private, for-profit ERCs than of institutional ERCs). But there are some safeguards to help protect ERCs from such a narrow interest in merely protecting their institution's legal liability. The most important of these safeguards is the quality and integrity of the persons who constitute these committees. (Guidelines for membership usually specifically exclude from participation in decision-making any person who might have a direct interest in a proposed protocol.[13]) Another safeguard is the Committee members' awareness of the need to maintain their moral credibility if their work is to carry any authority and is to be at all effective. In addition, the committees' structural autonomy from the research segments of the parent institutions, their dedication to continuing self-education, and the freedom with which they are able to make their decisions are all intended to best promote the committees' focus on protecting research subjects.

18.2 TWO LEVELS OF ETHICAL REVIEW

There is, however, some confusion in the mix of ethical questions that today's ERCs are asked to deal with. To help distinguish and clarify some of the complexities in this mix of ethical questions that ERCs are asked to weigh, I would propose that there be two separate levels of ethical review. My suggestion is the following: after a proposed human subjects protocol has gone through a scientific review, there should then be two separate levels of ethical review, and in the best case the two separate levels should be performed by two separate committees.

The first level of ethical review would focus primarily on protecting the interests and well-being of the individual subjects who will volunteer for these trials. This level would weigh the potential harms and benefits for the individual subjects, and would determine whether the trial had been designed in the best possible way to protect the subjects to the fullest extent possible, while at the same time effectively answering the scientific questions addressed by the study. This level would review issues of informed consent, autonomy, justice, and the balance of potential harms and benefits for subjects, just as today's ERCs do.

The second level of ethical review would come into play only after the protocol has passed both the scientific review and the first level of ethical review, and would ask an entirely separate set of ethical questions. It would ask whether this best possible trial – i.e., this trial which has been designed in the best possible way to both answer the scientific questions posed to it and to protect the human subjects who will volunteer for it – is ultimately ethically acceptable when you consider *all* the costs and *all* the benefits involved. It would probably be at this level that the considerations raised by Grady about community benefit would be examined and weighed.[14] Whereas the first level of ethical review would weigh harms and benefits, informed consent and justice for individual subjects in this particular trial, the second level of ethical review would weigh the total potential human costs (economic, social, psychological, etc.) against the total potential human benefits (knowledge to be gained, potential medical advances, potential reduction of human suffering, etc.). It may turn out to be the case, for example, that a given well designed trial simply should not be done, even though it is the most ethical trial that can be designed to answer the questions posed. It may be that weighing "the potential for scientific knowledge (against the consequences of not acquiring such information) and the financial, social, and human costs associated with conducting (or not conducting) such a trial,"[15] would result in a decision that undertaking the protocol would ultimately be unwise and unethical. That is to say, if the first level of ethical review would weigh harms against benefits for the individual subjects in the trials, this second level of review would weigh the total potential human costs against the total potential human gains for the whole community.

ERCs that perform the second level of ethical review would function in much the same capacity as the US national AIDS Research Advisory Committee (ARAC) functioned in May and June of 1994 when it weighed all the relevant factors for phase III trials of the Genentech and Chiron HIV subunit vaccines and decided to recommend that NIH not approve efficacy trials for these products in the US. This proposed second level of review would also be similar in purpose and scope to that of the WHO/GPA ad hoc committee which weighed the same type of candidate vaccine in October of 1994, and, contrary to the US committee opened the door for efficacy trials to be performed in one of three possible developing nations.[16] My proposal is that such second-level committees should not be ad hoc committees, but should instead be available to review all large-scale efficacy trials (particularly high-risk/low-benefit trials), and should be made up of a membership similar to the membership of present day ERCs, as to their distribution and representation.

A proposed protocol, therefore, would need to be approved at all three levels of review (in this sequence) before being funded and before being granted funding, time, space or facilities at any institution.

It is true that today's ERCs perform, to some degree, both of these separate review functions at the same time, but I believe the two different sets of questions, at the two different levels of ethical review, should be clearly distinguished from each other, and should be addressed separately. At the very least, today's ERCs should clearly distinguish between the two sets of ethical questions, and should address each of them separately, one after the other.

18.3 HIGH-RISK/LOW-BENEFIT PROTOCOLS

The CIOMS *Guidelines* do recognize that there may at times be a research protocol proposed which promises little if any benefit to individual subjects in the study, but great potential benefit to society at large, or promises a major increase in scientific knowledge. Research protocols of this sort, say the *Guidelines,* may be undertaken, but only under certain strictly defined narrow conditions. If research of this sort is ever to be undertaken, the *Guidelines* require that it not be done on subjects who are "members of vulnerable groups and persons with limited capacity to consent." Such research must instead involve only subjects "who are fully capable of [complete] informed consent and who understand and accept [all] the risks."[17]

In other words, in order that research sponsors not be even slightly tempted to take unfair advantage of potentially vulnerable populations, such high risk research must be done only with subjects who are completely capable of full awareness of all the risks attendant on their participation in the high risk trials, and who fully understand what these risks entail. We may seriously doubt whether many prospective subjects in some of the developing communities proposed for these vaccine trials would completely meet these specifications, particularly because of lower literacy and education rates, less familiarity with the concepts and procedures of modern medical practice, and possibly even completely different concepts of disease and disease causation than those held by the researchers. As one author says of African subjects (though it may apply to subjects in some other parts of the world as well):

> African subjects with relatively little understanding of medical aspects of research participation, indisposed toward resisting the suggestions of Western doctors, perhaps operating under the mistaken notion that they are being treated, and possibly receiving some ancillary benefits from participation in the research, are very susceptible to coercion [even if unintentional].[18]

Or if not susceptible to coercion (which seems a rather strong term), perhaps we should say that they are susceptible to accidental manipulation by researchers, even perhaps by researchers who have absolutely no conscious intentions of trying to manipulate anyone.

If it is true, therefore, to say that phase III HIV vaccine trials may indeed entail significant (or at least a large number of) risks for volunteers who would participate, and few if any benefits for them, then ERCs will have to decide a) if these vaccine trials should be considered to be high-risk/low-benefit protocols. If the trials should be considered as such, then ERCs will also have to decide b) whether sponsors should perform these trials among vulnerable populations in developing nations. If ERCs were to approve such trials in developing nations, then the Antithesis position would wonder whether those committees were meeting their primary responsibility of protecting the human subjects, particularly those human subjects who belong to potentially vulnerable populations?

These are difficult questions.

Even in the short history of the existence of ERCs late in the 20th century, it has already become increasingly evident how important the role of such committees has been and will probably continue to be, particularly in their role as protectors of research volunteers. It has also become evident how important it will be for ERCs to maintain their autonomy, their freedom of deliberation, their integrity of judgment, and their great good sense.

How such committees come into existence, how they are funded, how they are constituted, how they maintain their independence and autonomy, and how they proceed in their deliberations and decision-making are all issues of great consequence (they are also matters which vary considerably from committee to committee, and from institution to institution) but they are beyond the scope of this book. It should be clear, however, that these issues will have definite bearing on how decisions are made about phase III vaccine trials.

I will add only that, according to the CIOMS *Ethical Guidelines*, any ERC that reviews research protocols which will be performed in underdeveloped communities, whether those communities are in developed or developing nations, must have "among its members or consultants persons who are thoroughly familiar with the customs and traditions of the [developing] community" under consideration.[19] All seem to agree that this requirement is absolutely essential.

NOTES

1. E. D. Prentice, et al., "Bill of Rights for Research Subjects", *IRB, A Review of Human Subjects Research,* 15.2, March–April (1993) 7–9, p 7.
2. R. J. Levine. *Ethics and Regulation of Clinical Research.* Second ed. (New Haven, CT: Yale University Press, 1986, 1988) 452+xx, p 393.
3. 45 CFR 46.
4. 45 CFR 46, § 46.103, b, 1. R. J. Levine. *Ethics and Regulation of Clinical Research.* Second ed. (New Haven, CT: Yale University Press, 1986, 1988) 452+xx, p 397.
5. R. J. Levine. *Ethics and Regulation of Clinical Research.* Second ed. (New Haven, CT: Yale University Press, 1986, 1988) 452+xx, p 326.
6. G. J. Annas and M. A. Grodin, eds. *The Nazi Doctors and the Nuremberg Code: Human Rights in Human Experimentation.* (New York, NY: Oxford University Press, 1992) 371+xxii, pp 267–68.
7. I. Kant. *Fundamental Principles of the Metaphysic of Morals.* Trans. Thomas Kingsmill Abbott. vol. 42 of 54, (Chicago, IL: The Great Books of the Western World, Encyclopedia Britannica, Inc, 1785, 1952), p 272.
8. Quoted in D. J. Rothman. *Strangers at the Bedside: A history of how law and bioethics transformed medical decision making* (Basic Books, Harper Collins, 1991) 303+xii, p 23.

   Bernard does, however, add one more sentence which makes this dictum a bit more ambiguous: " . . . and so among the experiments that may be tried on man, those that can only harm are forbidden, and those that may do good are obligatory." Quoted in C. Grady RN, PhD. *The Search for an AIDS Vaccine* of (Indianapolis, IN: Indiana University Press, 1995) 193, p 32.
9. D. Hodel and AIDS Action Foundation Working Group. *HIV Preventive Vaccines: Social, Ethical, and Political Considerations* (AIDS Action Foundation, Office of AIDS Research, National Institutes of Health, 1994), p 23.
10. E. Kessel, "Estimating Risks and Benefits in AIDS Vaccine and Drug Trials," *AIDS & Public Policy Journal,* 5,4, Winter (1990) 186–88.
11. N. A. Christakis, "The Ethical Design of an AIDS Vaccine Trial in Africa," *Hastings Center Report,* 18, 3, June/July (1988) 31–37, p 35.
12. C. Grady RN, PhD. *The Search for an AIDS Vaccine* (Indianapolis, IN: Indiana University Press, 1995) 193, pp 64–66, 83–85.
13. R. J. Levine. "AIDS Research and Ethical Review Boards." *Ethics and Law in the Study of AIDS.* Eds. H. Fuenzalida-Puelma, A. M. L. Parada

and D. S. LaVertu (Washington, D C: Pan American Health Organization, Regional Office of the World Health Organization, 1992) 170–77, p 171.

14. C. Grady RN, PhD. *The Search for an AIDS Vaccine* (Indianapolis, IN: Indiana University Press, 1995) 193.
15. D. Hodel and AIDS Action Foundation Working Group. *HIV Preventive Vaccines: Social, Ethical, and Political Considerations* AIDS Action Foundation, Office of AIDS Research, National Institutes of Health, 1994), p 1.
16. See the Reuters news story of October 14, 1994 to which I referred in the Introduction.
17. Commentary on Guideline 14, Z. Bankowski. *International Ethical Guidelines for Biomedical Research Involving Human Subjects* (Geneva, Switzerland: Council for International Organizations of Medical Sciences (CIOMS), 1993) 63, p 39.

    For an argument supporting this position, see also A. R. Jonsen, "The Ethics of Using Human Volunteers for High-Risk Research," *Journal of Infectious Diseases*, 160 August (1989) 205–208.
18. N. A. Christakis, "The Ethical Design of an AIDS Vaccine Trial in Africa," *Hastings Center Report*, 18, 3 June/July (1988) 31–37, p 35.
19. Z. Bankowski, ed. *International Ethical Guidelines for Biomedical Research Involving Human Subjects*. (Geneva, Switzerland: Council for International Organizations of Medical Sciences (CIOMS), 1993) 63, Guideline 8, p 25.

    Carol Levine, et al. add one more similar suggestion discussed by their working group:

    "IRBs that regularly review HIV/AIDS research should seriously consider including among their members representatives of or advocates for populations of prospective subjects and intended beneficiaries." C. Levine, N. N. Dubler and R. J. Levine, "Building a New Consensus: Ethical Principles and Policies for Clinical Research on HIV/AIDS," *IRB*, 13, 1–2 January–April (1991) 1–17, p 11.

    This suggestion was controversial in the discussions of this working group, but it might be less controversial if the suggestion applied only to the times that an ERC is considering AIDS related research.

19 Proxy Consent?

Sponsors of phase III HIV vaccine trials in developing nations may ask to be excused from the requirement to fully inform each individual prospective subject and to obtain each individual prospective subject's free and uncoerced consent. They could base their request on the difficulty (or impossibility) of explaining such complex material to persons in communities with less than optimum literacy, and/or on the length of time it would take to so educate each individual subject. They might also base their request on the perceived difficulty of finding large numbers of persons who are "so situated as to be able to exercise free power of choice," i.e., who are completely free of any possibility of coercion, constraint, duress, or intimidation. That is, they could ask instead to invoke the principle of proxy consent.

If research sponsors do ask to resort to proxies for consent, using perhaps tribal chiefs, military officers, or local health officials, as they have often done in the past,[1] then those proxies will have to possess certain qualifications. The ERC will doubtless require that those who would be proxies a) be competent[2] to make reasoned judgments, b) have adequate knowledge and information on which to base their judgments, c) have emotional stability, and d) have a commitment to the "incompetent" subjects' interests, which is "free of conflicts of interest and free of controlling influence by others who may not seek the [subject's] best interests."[3]

It would probably not be difficult to find proxies who would meet qualification a) and c), i.e., who are legally competent and emotionally stable. It may be more difficult, however, to find proxies who will have adequate knowledge and information about all the various aspects of HIV vaccine trials. And it might be even more difficult to find proxies who would satisfy condition d), i.e., who are completely free of conflicts of interest, particularly if they are in positions of influence and power. In the case of army recruits, for example, finding a proxy who has a commitment to the subjects' best interests and well being may take some doing.

Even if such proxies could be found, and even if such proxies could be adequately informed and educated about the risks (and benefits?) to volunteers who participate in this research, there is still the task of insuring that these proxies are not subject to coercion, to undue influence, or to undue inducement.

NOTES

1. L. K. Altman MD. "After Setback, First Large AIDS Vaccine Trials Are Planned." *New York Times* November 29 1994, B6.
2. A competent individual is one "who has received the necessary information; who has adequately understood the information; and who, after considering the information, has arrived at a decision without having been subjected to coercion, undue influence or inducement, or intimidation." Z. Bankowski and R. J. Levine, eds. *Ethics and Research on Human Subjects: International Guidelines (Proceedings of the XXVIth CIOMS Conference, Geneva, Switzerland, 5–7 February 1992)* (Geneva, Switzerland: Council for International Organizations of Medical Sciences (CIOMS), 1993) 228+63+x, p 13, Commentary for Guideline 1.
3. T. L. Beauchamp and J. F. Childress. *Principles of Biomedical Ethics.* Third ed. (New York: Oxford University Press, 1989) 470+x, p 178.

20 Undue Inducement

Ethicists agree that the informed consent given by subjects must be free and uncoerced. The first paragraph in section I of *The Nuremberg Code* says specifically that

> the person involved should be so situated as to be able to exercise free power of choice, without the intervention of any element of force, fraud, deceit, duress, overreaching, or other ulterior form of constraint or coercion.[1]

To what extent can this be insured in developing nations where trials are conducted? Consider 21 year old Royal Thai Army recruits, for example, or 19 year old Ugandan army recruits. Or consider injection drug users and their (to some degree) desperate physiological need for their next fix, and for the money to pay for it. Are these persons "so situated as to be able to exercise free power of choice," as *The Nuremberg Code* requires? Might it be that they would be subject to some forms of force or duress with regard to their proposed participation in vaccine trials? Should injection drug users, for example, be asked for their consent when they are sober, to insure that they are not under the influence of an intoxicant?[2] Or should they be asked for their consent after they have had a fix, when they might be considered to be less subject to manipulation by those who would like them to consent? (Physicians who specialize in the practice of addiction medicine are clearly the experts who need to be consulted on questions of this sort, as well as other questions related to the participation of IDUs in these trials.) These are not easy questions. Those who design these protocols will need to be mindful of these difficulties.

Besides insuring that subjects have not been in any degree coerced into giving their consent, researchers must also be on guard against undue influence and undue inducements to participate. An inducement, according to medical ethicists,

> consists of an offer to a person of something of value in exchange for his or her agreement to do something that

he or she might not do without the inducement. A simple example of an inducement is a cash payment. A cash payment so large that it overwhelms other relevant considerations – e.g., risk/benefit assessment – in the decision to be or to continue to be a research subject is called an "undue inducement."[3]

The issue of undue inducement is addressed in Guideline 4 of *The International Ethical Guidelines.*

> Subjects may be paid for inconvenience and time spent, and should be reimbursed for expenses incurred, in connection with their participation in research; they may also receive free medical services. However, the payments should not be so large or the medical services so extensive as to induce prospective subjects to consent to participate in the research against their better judgment ("undue inducement").[4]

Undue inducement to participate is unethical and invalidates free consent, according to virtually all writing on the subject. The Commentary on Guideline 4 says that "payments in money or in kind to research subjects should not be so large as to persuade them to take undue risk or volunteer against their better judgment."[5] Furthermore,

> It may be difficult to distinguish between suitable recompense and undue influence to participate in research. An unemployed person or a student may view promised recompense differently from an employed person. Someone without access to medical care may be unduly influenced to participate in research simply to receive such care.[6]

In some underdeveloped communities, almost *any* payment, and almost *any* medical care, might constitute "undue recompense," if economic standards in the community are very low. In some communities it will be difficult, perhaps almost impossible, for researchers to satisfy the requirement to avoid undue inducement. If they cannot fully satisfy that ethical requirement, what then? Would that be a violation of the *International Ethical Guidelines,* or of the section of *The Nuremberg Code* which requires that all subjects be "so situated as to be able to exercise free power of choice?"

These too are difficult questions.

NOTES

1. See Appendix I.
2. One author suggests, for example, that "Active drug users must be recruited only when sober so that they can fully understand the nature of the study." D. F. Hoth, et al., "HIV Vaccine Development: A Progress Report," *Annals of Internal Medicine,* 8, 7, 15 October (1994) 603–11, p 609.
3. C. Levine, N. N. Dubler and R. J. Levine, "Building a New Consensus: Ethical Principles and Policies for Clinical Research on HIV/AIDS," *IRB,* 13, 1–2, January–April (1991) 1–17, p 13.
4. Z. Bankowski, ed. *International Ethical Guidelines for Biomedical Research Involving Human Subjects* (Geneva, Switzerland: Council for International Organizations of Medical Sciences (CIOMS), 1993) 63, Guideline 4, p 18.
5. Other examples of undue inducement "would be to induce a close relative or a community leader to influence a prospective subject's decision or to threaten to withhold health services." Z. Bankowski, ed. *International Guidelines for Ethical Review of Epidemiological Studies* (Geneva: World Health Organization, 1991), p 17.
6. *Ibid.*, p. 19.

21 Motivations to Volunteer

If research sponsors must avoid undue inducement in order to avoid the problem of invalidating "free consent," then another question begins to surface: why would anyone choose to volunteer as a subject in these vaccine studies? The risks involved would seem to provide good reasons for some potential volunteers to decline participation. In addition, general feelings of distrust toward government agencies (who would probably be co-sponsoring such studies) is hardly a peculiarity of Western societies. In the US, the history of ethically questionable medical experimentation, such as the Tuskegee study of untreated syphilis in black men, as well as numerous instances of government insensitivity toward persons of color, has made it exceptionally difficult for vaccine researchers to recruit black volunteers.[1] Researchers in some AIDS Vaccine Evaluation Units around the US, for example, have had a difficult time convincing members of the black community that this time, in this research, for this sexually transmitted disease, the government is going to treat them fairly and ethically. A study of 1160 gay men in Denver, San Francisco and Chicago found that 86 per cent of them had serious misgivings about how much the government could be trusted, or had "a real fear about the government."[2] It would not surprise me to learn that Ugandans, whose recent history has included Idi Amin and a number of other oppressive dictators, have similar feelings of distrust toward government agencies. If Brazilians and Thais sometimes have similar distrust of government, then whatever would motivate persons to volunteer as subjects in a vaccine trial that had been reviewed, approved, and recommended by the government, given this potential distrust and these real risks? Are there any good reasons an ordinary citizen might have for offering to volunteer in these trials? Some possible motivations do come to mind.

21.1 ALTRUISM

Altruism is probably the real motivation for some volunteers. Such volunteers will probably be very aware of the seriousness of the pandemic and will want to do something to help out. Perhaps their brother or daughter died of AIDS in recent months or years, and by volunteering as a subject in a vaccine study they perhaps feel they can somehow express their love for him or her, and at the same time try to do something to help fight the epidemic, and perhaps even benefit the wider human community. Particularly in phase I trials, in which subjects need to be seronegative (as is necessary for all three phases of the trials), and must not be at any significant degree of risk for becoming infected with HIV (as phase III volunteers must be), altruism seems so far to be the main motivator. Phase I studies require only a small number of subjects (approximately 30–80), and it may not be difficult to find this number of persons who are willing to volunteer, at some risk to themselves, and for virtually no benefit, just because they want to help out. But researchers for phase II trials which require a larger number of subjects, and phase III trials which require thousands, or tens of thousands, of subjects, may have difficulty finding a large enough number of people who will volunteer for purely humanitarian reasons, in spite of the risks and with no particular benefit to themselves.

So we need to ask what benefits a volunteer might imagine would accrue to them which could outweigh the risks he or she faces by joining one of these studies? Some possible perceived benefits might include the following.

21.2 MONEY

Money paid to them by researchers might be a sufficient motivation for some volunteers, but the amount of that money must be extremely negligible, otherwise it would violate the undue inducement clauses of the *International Ethical Guidelines.* In some communities, in order to protect against even the appearance of undue inducement, the amount of money paid to volunteers will need to be very small indeed.

21.3 MEDICAL CARE

The promise of medical care may be an incentive for some, but the extent of that medical care will need to be extremely minimal, otherwise that too will constitute undue inducement. It seems clear that the *Guidelines* proscribe both money and medical care, except in minimal amounts, as prime incentives to participate in the research. So lacking these motivators, are there any other reasons that might incline a person to participate in such a vaccine study?

21.4 THE CHANCE OF PROTECTION

One possible incentive for a volunteer to participate in a vaccine trial is their belief that they might be lucky, that they could be one of the random subjects who actually gets the candidate vaccine rather than the placebo, that the candidate vaccine they get might be a relatively safe and effective one, and that they could therefore be protected, to some degree, from getting infected with HIV or contracting AIDS.[3] Since this may in fact be the motivation of many potential volunteers, the preliminary education and informing of potential subjects, before they volunteer, will need to make some important points very clear:

1. It must be made clear that the "vaccine" being studied is only *possibly* an effective vaccine, that it is not known whether this candidate vaccine will be effective at all, and that therefore the candidate vaccine should not be relied on to protect anyone from anything.
2. It must also be made clear that this study is a placebo-controlled study, which means that only a certain percent of subjects will receive the actual candidate vaccine, and that all other subjects (perhaps 30–50 per cent)[4] will receive only an inert placebo which has no effect of any sort and confers no protection against anything. (Another question for ethicists to consider: should potential volunteers also be told the exact percentage of probability that they will receive the candidate vaccine or the placebo, so they can calculate their chances?)

3 It must also be made clear that even if they do happen to receive the candidate vaccine and even if it does prove to be effective to some extent, it would still probably be effective only a certain per cent of the time. In other words, it must be stressed that no vaccine, not even the very best, is anywhere near 100 per cent effective, and that present HIV candidate vaccines will probably be very much less effective – perhaps only 30–60 per cent effective – than most vaccines already in existence for other diseases.
4 Finally, it must be stressed that during the entire study subjects will be counseled and urged to *not* engage in any behaviors that put them at risk of HIV infection. In other words, pre-study educators will have a strong obligation to make it clear that subjects would be foolish to rely on whatever they receive in this study to protect them from HIV infection.

Nevertheless, in spite of such pre-trial counseling and informing, some potential subjects may feel that a very small chance of some small degree of protection is better than no chance at all. These potential subjects may be planning to continue their risky behaviors, and may therefore see participation in a vaccine study as an opportunity to increase their chances for survival, even if by only a small percentage. These subjects, of course, are the very ones who, because they will feel safer, may even *increase* their risk behaviors, and thereby worsen their chances of infection, and possibly even worsen the spread of the epidemic. Nevertheless, unrealistic and unwise as their thinking may be in this matter, the possibility of getting protected may well be some subjects' motivation for participating in the trials.

21.5 OTHER MOTIVES

Other motives to participate may include a desire to be seen as a good community member, or a desire to think of oneself as forwarding the aims of scientific research, or even a desire to do one more good act (by being a research subject) despite continuing to participate in risky behaviors.

Some persons may volunteer simply because they were told to do so by a boss, a spouse, a partner, a community leader, or military officer. They may have even been threatened, and hence forced to volunteer. Others may volunteer because of having experienced a great deal of social pressure to volunteer. The consent of these "volunteers," of course, would thus have been coerced, and therefore ethically invalid, but the coercion may be completely invisible to (i.e., hidden from) those who are conducting the trial.

Some form of "easy out" should probably be offered to all prospective subjects just to avoid this possible eventuality. For example, when a local blood center has a blood drive seeking voluntary donations of blood, a certain office group or boss may decide that the whole office staff should go together and donate blood. If one person in the office is HIV+, and hence should not donate any blood, but is afraid to disclose that fact to his or her coworkers, that person may feel forced to go along with the group and donate his or her blood anyhow, just to protect their privacy. Fortunately, blood banks have provided an "easy out" just for persons in situations like this. When a person is filling out his or her donor card, there is a little box at the bottom of the card that says "Do not use this blood for any purposes." If you check that box (you need not give any explanation, and they will not ask for any), then they will not use your blood; they will throw it away. They will, however, go through all the motions of drawing your blood just as they are drawing everyone else's blood, and you will have given the full appearance of having participated in the office blood drive, thus protecting your confidentiality. To all appearances, you donated blood just as everyone else did.

It may be wise to provide an "easy out" of this same sort for any volunteers who might need it. They would then be able to avoid actual participation in the trial, but would be able to give the impression that they had volunteered to participate.

It seems that some of the potential motivations reviewed above are probably not well thought out, and hence might not be sufficient motivation to sustain a subject throughout the whole course of a study. Other motivations, such as altruism, may not motivate a large enough number of subjects. Research sponsors will doubtless want to have it clear in their own minds what sorts of reasons would motivate subjects to participate in their protocols. In some communities, finding volunteers for the studies may require a certain amount of active marketing. If that turns out to be the case, another whole set of ethical considerations will need to be discussed and implemented concerning the methods and procedures for carrying out such marketing and advertising.

21.6 QUITTING

Volunteers will remember that they have been told clearly and directly by research sponsors that they can drop out of the study at any time they wish, without incurring any cost or penalty. Whatever motivation they may have for participating, therefore, will have to be enough of a motivation to sustain them throughout the long months and years that the trial lasts. It is no small inconvenience to researchers when subjects choose to quit the study, since research sponsors will have invested a good amount of time, effort, and financial resources in each volunteer. When one volunteer quits it may mean having to recruit another, with all the time and cost that would entail, and, if a large number of subjects quit the trial, it may even mean a consequent postponement of the trial's termination date. Trial sponsors will not want to have subjects quitting the study. But on the other hand, subjects must be made aware that they are allowed to quit at any time they wish for any reason at all (or even for no reason).

I have been told of some vaccine research protocols that asked volunteers to sign a "commitment form" when they join the study. This practice seems to me to be designed for the benefit of the research sponsors rather than for the benefit of the research subjects. I have privately wondered how ERCs that reviewed those protocols might have justified the requirement for subjects to sign a commitment form, in light of the requirement that each volunteer be made fully aware that they can quit the study at any time for any reason.

Having considered these possible motivations for why some persons might choose to join and stay in a vaccine study, we could now find ourselves wondering whether these motivations will be sufficient, either for the subjects or for the sponsors. We will not know the answer to this question, despite some recent studies that try to assess the future motivations and behaviors of certain groups, until recruitment programs for the trials actually begin.

NOTES

1. E. Blackstone, personal communication about UW's vaccine studies, 22 July 1994.
2. D. Hodel and AIDS Action Foundation Working Group. *HIV Preventive Vaccines: Social, Ethical, and Political Considerations* (AIDS Action Foundation, Office of AIDS Research, National Institutes of Health, 1994), p 8.
3. Christakis believes this should be considered a benefit to individual subjects. He says: "The salient personal benefit to participation in an AIDS vaccine trial is the possibility of gaining immunity to a deadly infection." N. A. Christakis, "The Ethical Design of an AIDS Vaccine Trial in Africa," *Hastings Center Report*, 18, 3, June/July (1988) 31–37, p 33.
4. Dr José Esparza, director of the HIV vaccine effort at the WHO, estimates that a likely phase III HIV vaccine trial may entail "a three-arm trial, one placebo and one each of the two candidate vaccines, with 9000 subjects in a place with a high incidence of HIV infection." He estimates that such a trial in a developing nation may cost approximately $45 million. Cotton, "International Disunity on HIV Vaccine Efficacy Trials," *JAMA*, 272, 14.12, October (1994) 190–91, p 1091.

22 Still More Questions

As if the questions we have been asking so far have not been problematic enough, still more questions come to mind, especially in the minds of those who hold the Antithesis position. Among these questions are the following:

> Is it truly realistic, especially in developing nations, to expect that researchers and sponsors will actually comply with these ethical guidelines? Won't researchers be tempted to cut ethical corners? Might it even be possible that Ethics Review Committees will not actually require strict adherence to CIOMS *Guidelines*, but instead will require researchers only to "make a reasonable effort" to comply with the guidelines?

If this were to happen, the results could be disastrous for the research sponsors and for the future of the vaccine trials. Such ethical laxity could run the serious risk of actually, in the long run, completely derailing a research protocol, and setting back for years the possible development of a successful vaccine.

In fact, if such ethical laxity were to come to pass, could it not happen that twenty years from now we would all be looking back – as today we look back on the Willowbrook hepatitis study, on the Tuskegee syphilis study, and on the experiments observing the effects of close-range nuclear radiation on human beings – that we would all be looking back with condemnation at scandalous human experiments that were perpetrated upon masses of innocent and vulnerable peoples in developing nations? Could it be that we will be watching *20/20* exposés of large pharmaceutical companies, and large Western government agencies, exploiting naive and desperate (and inexpensive) peoples in lesser developed countries? Could it happen that historians will be appalled that one of the reasons pharmaceutical companies wanted to do research in underdeveloped communities was because it was less expensive to do the research there, where subjects were pliable and ready at hand, and where labor was cheap?[1] Could it be that we will discover that their bottom line was profit, and not the benefit of the human species?

Or instead might it be that we will discover in retrospect that these were times of courage and heroism, times in which many individuals and even some governments were committed to discovering a vaccine that would help the world contain a plague which threatened to do immense damage to human society?

Whichever scenario turns out to be closer to reality will depend largely on the work of those who sponsor, design, and implement these phase III vaccine protocols. It will also depend on the work of ethicists who examine the principles that apply in such trials, and on the work of Ethics Review Committees which will be examining in minute detail each protocol brought before them.

The four main questions these ERCs will be asking are:

1 Is this proposed protocol scientifically sound? Has it undergone a thorough scientific review and has it been determined that there is solid scientific justification for going ahead with this study? Are all the investigators involved competent to be overseeing, directing or participating in the study? Is the design of the protocol sufficient to meet, in Robert Levine's terms, "the nearly universal standards of the relevant scientific discipline."[2] This scientific review process is normally done well before the ethical review, so the ERC will have some solid data to review on this score.

ERCs will ask, for example, some of the following questions: have researchers satisfied themselves that HIV truly is the significant etiologic agent against which we must vaccinate? (See Chapter 5, Section 5.1 above on the question of etiologicity.) Do laboratory and animal studies provide strong evidence that this vaccine will protect against more than one strain of the virus, and that it will last for more than a few months? Are researchers convinced that the vaccine will probably not cause more harm than good? Are they confident that HIV will not simply mutate its way around this vaccine? Have researchers faced the issues of the emerging "Darwinian medicine?" Have they dealt with the issues surrounding the evolution of virulence?

Also, have researchers determined whether the criterion of vaccine success is prevention of infection (an almost impossibly high and strict criterion of success), prevention of disease (the most historically common criterion of success in vaccines for other infectious diseases), postponement of disease, or attenuation of disease (more modest, and perhaps more realistic, criteria of success)?[3]

Furthermore, is the actual design of the protocol scientifically sound? Have researchers adequately isolated the significant variables? Is the protocol sufficiently double-blinded and randomized? Is there a control group of adequate size and randomness? Have sponsors clarified how long the study will last, and are their reasons for choosing that time period sound?

An ethics committee's interest in these questions will not be cursory or perfunctory. The reason for an ERC's interest in questions of scientific methodology is that for a sponsor to initiate a human subjects study without a sound scientific foundation is *ipso facto* a serious breach of ethical principles, most importantly because it may expose subjects to inconvenience and risk for no sound purpose.[4] A poorly designed study could end up being all risk and no benefit to anyone at all. As Robert Levine so clearly states,

> [T]he requirement for good research design is an ethical requirement. Moreover, it is a requirement of such importance that it must be satisfied first. If it cannot be satisfied, there is no need to consider such other requirements as informed consent or equitable selection of subjects.[5]

In addition, a poorly designed trial, i.e., one that failed to adequately answer the scientific question, "is a waste of precious time and resources, both human and economic."[6]

2 The second kind of question ERCs will ask is whether there is an acceptable and proportionate potential-harm to potential-benefit ratio for each individual research subject. This is one of the most important questions ERCs ask and it is taken very seriously.[7] Yet, in HIV vaccine trials, one is hard pressed to find anything that could be

counted as a direct *benefit* to individual volunteers.[8] What might they gain from participating in this research that could possibly balance the amount of risk they are undertaking? Will they be paid for their trouble? Will they be given free medical care? Yes, of course, but they will not be paid very much, or given very much medical care, because that would violate the proscription against undue inducement.

The only thing that might really be called a benefit for the individual volunteers is the provision that "the population in which the vaccine is tested is entitled to first priority in receiving the vaccine after its safety and efficacy have been established."[9] If such a vaccine is proven safe and effective, it must be provided to these populations (and particularly to those vaccine research subjects who received the placebo vaccine) at minimal or no cost.

> It is considered essential that a vaccine or vaccines developed or evaluated through international scientific collaboration be made available to developing countries under the most advantageous possible conditions.[10]

This is a benefit, of course, but it is more a benefit to population groups than it is to individual subjects.[11] In addition, this benefit, if it ever did come to pass, would not be available for a good many years. Some subjects participating in these trials would probably not still be alive to enjoy this benefit.

It might be a bit of a stretch, therefore, (the Antithesis position will argue) to claim that there is any proportionate balance of risks and benefits for volunteers participating in these vaccine trials.

Yet this is considered one of the essential requirements in an ethically sound human subjects research protocol.

3 A third question ERCs will ask is whether investigators will realistically be able to protect their subjects against significant harm, whether that harm be physical, psychological or social.

The World Medical Association, meeting for the 41st World Medical Assembly in Hong Kong, in 1989, amended and reaffirmed the Declaration of Helsinki of 1964. This declaration is a set of recommendations for "guiding physicians in biomedical research involving human subjects." Its principles provided the foundation for the CIOMS document we have been examining in this book. The recommendations are very clear about the obligation of researchers to protect the wellbeing of subjects who participate in their research:

> In . . . medical research carried out on a human being, it is the duty of the physician to remain the protector of the life and health of that person on whom biomedical research is being carried out.[12]

These recommendations emphasize that this is particularly applicable in those research protocols (such as HIV vaccine trials) which have no therapeutic purposes, i.e., which are not intended to cure anything. These same recommendations also emphasize that the individual rights of volunteers must always take higher precedence than any social or scientific benefit that might be foreseen. "In research on man," says this document, "the interest of science and society should never take precedence over considerations related to the wellbeing of the [individual research] subject."[13]

Ethics committees will therefore be asking how well researchers and their sponsors will be able to protect their subjects against the kinds of hazards – physical, social, psychological, and economic – described above in Chapter 11.

Those who hold the Antithesis position may have serious doubts.

4 Will investigators be able to obtain every single subject's properly informed and freely given consent? We have seen ways in which this may prove to be quite difficult.

In reflecting on some of these impossibly difficult ethical issues facing HIV vaccine trials in developing nations, some intelligent yet frustrated readers may find themselves almost desperately hoping for some larger and simpler solution to this whole tangle of ethical and research problems. "Maybe we will never even have to do vaccine trials after all. Maybe some other solution to the AIDS problem will come to us from the genetics researchers, or from the recombinant DNA laboratories, or from NASA's studies of how life forms procreate in gravity-free conditions. Or from *any*where. *Some*where. Please!"

While such a fantasized solution would be something devoutly to be wished, there is nothing on the visible horizon to inspire any realistic soul's feeling of hopefulness in this direction. Creative solutions of all sorts should be imagined and sought, of course, but we would not be wise to hold our breath waiting for them.

"Or maybe," thinks our hypothetically frustrated reader, "maybe we should just not do vaccine trials in developing nations at all. Maybe we should just do the research on populations here in (insert 'the UK,' or 'France,' or 'the US') instead."

There is a certain altruistic and self-sacrificing spirit in such a reaction, as well as a commendable desire to avoid even the appearance of exploiting vulnerable peoples. But there are two serious problems with this "solution."

The first problem is that, even if we could avoid testing vaccines in developing nations, we would still have to test them in vulnerable and disadvantaged populations somewhere. Why? Because these are the groups that are disproportionately at high risk for infection with HIV, and therefore they are the groups that need a vaccine the most.[14] If we want to develop a vaccine that will work for anybody, we want one that will work for the vulnerable and oppressed peoples of the earth, i.e., for those people most at risk and most in need of a vaccine. If a vaccine will ever work for them, then at some point it must be tested on them.

The second problem with that imagined solution is that there are a wide variety of strains of HIV, and there are significantly different strains in different parts of the world. There are also different modes of transmission,[15] different endemic diseases and other underlying health problems, potentially significant genetic differences,[16] and different microbiological ecologies in different regions of the world. If we did not test vaccines in any developing nations, we would probably not end up with a vaccine that would be effective against the strains of HIV, and its modes of transmission, predominant in those countries. As the CIOMS *Guidelines* make clear

> [M]odes of transmission of the infection, and the natural history of the disease, may differ substantially among communities. Moreover, strains of HIV are different in various regions of the world, and the current scientific understanding is that different strains may respond differently to vaccines or drugs. If research were conducted only in developed countries and communities, developing countries could be deprived of many of the benefits of such research.[17]

In other words, *not* testing candidate vaccines in the populations most at risk would also be a serious ethical blunder.

NOTES

1. "Under the principle of justice, research subjects should be chosen 'for reasons directly related to the problem being studied,' and not 'because of their easy availability, their compromised position, or their manipulability.' Thus the practical concerns that make an AIDS vaccine trial easier to conduct in Africa do not alone constitute sufficient justification to use Africans as subjects. Only the scientific concerns related directly to the problem of establishing the ability of a vaccine to prevent HIV infection are relevant." N. A. Christakis, "The Ethical Design of an AIDS Vaccine Trial in Africa," *Hastings Center Report,* 18, 3, June/July (1988) 31–37, p 36. The quoted sections of this passage are taken from *The Belmont Report: Ethical Principles and Guidelines for the Protection of Human Subjects of Research.* National Commission for the Protection of Human Subjects of Biomedican and Behavioral Research, Department of Health, Education and Welfare, 1979, p 5.
2. R. J. Levine. "AIDS Research and Ethical Review Boards." *Ethics and Law in the Study of AIDS.* Eds. H. Fuenzalida-Puelma, A. M. L. Parada and D. S. LaVertu (Washington, DC: Pan American Health Organization, Regional Office of the World Health Organization, 1992) 170–77, p 172.
3. "In humans, vaccination might attenuate the course of the illness in cases in which it failed actually to prevent infection." M. D. Grmek MD, PhD. *History of AIDS: Emergence and Origin of a Modern Pandemic.* Trans. Maulitz, Russell, and Duffin, Jacalyn (Princeton, NJ: Princeton University Press, 1990) 279+xii, p 187.

4. "Scientific review and ethical review cannot be clearly separated: scientifically unsound research on human subjects is *ipso facto* unethical in that it may expose subjects to risk or inconvenience to no purpose. Normally, therefore, ethical review committees consider both the scientific and the ethical aspects of proposed research." Z. Bankowski, ed. *International Ethical Guidelines for Biomedical Research Involving Human Subjects.* (Geneva, Switzerland: Council for International Organizations of Medical Sciences (CIOMS), 1993) 63, p 38.
5. R. J. Levine. "AIDS Research and Ethical Review Boards." *Ethics and Law in the Study of AIDS.* Eds. H. Fuenzalida-Puelma, A. M. L. Parada and D. S. LaVertu (Washington, DC: Pan American Health Organization, Regional Office of the World Health Organization, 1992) 170–77, pp 171–72.
6. D. Hodel and AIDS Action Foundation Working Group. *HIV Preventive Vaccines: Social, Ethical, and Political Considerations* (AIDS Action Foundation, Office of AIDS Research, National Institutes of Health, 1994), p 10.
7. T. L. Beauchamp and J. F. Childress. *Principles of Biomedical Ethics.* Third ed. (New York: Oxford University Press, 1989) 470+x, p 384.
8. A major preliminary study of ethical issues in HIV vaccine trials also seems to find few if any benefits to be gained by those who would volunteer for the trials. D. Hodel and AIDS Action Foundation Working Group. *HIV Preventive Vaccines: Social, Ethical, and Political Considerations* (AIDS Action Foundation, Office of AIDS Research, National Institutes of Health, 1994).
9. Global Programme on AIDS. *Statement from the Consultation on Criteria for International Testing of Candidate HIV Vaccines* (Geneva: World Health Organization, 1989) 13, p 3.
10. *Ibid.* p 10.
11. "Should an HIV vaccine be successfully developed, sponsors are obligated to provide access to volunteers who participated in trials – maximum advantage must then be accorded to those at highest risk for infection, without regard to their ability to pay." D. Hodel and AIDS Action Foundation Working Group. *HIV Preventive Vaccines: Social, Ethical, and Political Considerations* (AIDS Action Foundation, Office of AIDS Research, National Institutes of Health, 1994), p 27.

    Nevertheless, even though this recommendation is that individual volunteers be provided with any successful vaccine that is developed, if such vaccines are not licensed for ten or fifteen or twenty more years, it will probably be of small benefit to today's research participants.

    Furthermore, it will be of no benefit at all even to the society in which the trial was done "unless there is a financial commitment by the developed world to provide the vaccine." N. A. Christakis, "The Ethical Design of an AIDS Vaccine Trial in Africa," *Hastings Center Report,* 18, 3, June/July (1988) 31–37, p 36.

    On the other hand, consider Grady's argument, referred to earlier, that benefits to the community *should* be entered into the risk/benefit equation. C. Grady RN, PhD. *The Search for an AIDS Vaccine*

(Indianapolis, IN: Indiana University Press, 1995) 193.
12. Z. Bankowski, ed. *International Ethical Guidelines for Biomedical Research Involving Human Subjects* (Geneva, Switzerland: Council for International Organizations of Medical Sciences (CIOMS), 1993) 63, p 50. See also p 10.
13. *Ibid.* p 50.
14. As one author from Haiti says: "You must give us the tools to carry on this fight. The clinical trials must be done where they are most needed: the developing countries. Vaccines represent the only viable alternative. . . ." J. W. Pape et. al., "The Urge for an AIDS Vaccine: Perspectives from a Developing Country," *AIDS Research and Human Retroviruses*, 8, 8 (1992) 1535–37, p 1536.
15. One significant problem with some candidate vaccines is that they may be successful (to some degree) in protecting against HIV transmission via one route of infection – rectal transmission, for example – but not successful in protecting against HIV transmission via another route of infection – vaginal transmission, for example. It will be important to test candidate vaccines in groups exposed to a variety of transmission modes. B. D. Schoub. *AIDS & HIV in Perspective* (New York, NY: Cambridge University Press, 1994) 268+xx, p 196.
16. W. L. Heyward, et al., "Preparation for Phase III HIV vaccine efficacy trials: methods for the determination of HIV incidence," *AIDS*, 8, 9, September (1994) 1285–91, p 1289.
17. Z. Bankowski, ed. *International Ethical Guidelines for Biomedical Research Involving Human Subjects* (Geneva, Switzerland: Council for International Organizations of Medical Sciences (CIOMS), 1993) 63, p 28.

23 Data from Unethical Experiments?

These ethical questions are given even more consequence by the concern about what to do with data which has been garnered from experiments that are judged to be clearly unethical. This question has been an important one since the doctors' trials at Nuremberg. We might imagine, for example, a researcher today, whose protocol had been declined by an ERC in the country of origin, simply deciding to take that same protocol to a different part of the world where there are no formal requirements for ethical review, or at least where there are much less strict requirements, and there simply conducting the research outside the purview of strict ethical oversight. In this situation, a protocol that has been formally judged ethically inadequate might still manage to be conducted and to gather some data. What should be done with the data garnered from that experiment?

This question is not altogether hypothetical. Consider the following story which appeared in the press in September 1995, dateline Bombay, India.

> Indian health authorities are investigating reports that a US-based foundation illegally tested a new AIDS vaccine on people in Bombay and Calcutta.
>
> A World Health Organization official at an AIDS conference in Thailand yesterday condemned the reported tests, saying the vaccine had not even been used on animals.[1]

Suppose that such a vaccine study, judged to be scientifically and ethically questionable (at best), does manage to generate some amount of data. The question we are now considering is: how should the scientific community respond to data garnered from that experiment?

One suggestion has been to treat that data in the same way that the scientific community treats data garnered from experiments which are simply badly designed scientifically.

The data are simply ignored. This proposal, then, recommends that a protocol which has been judged ethically inadequate should also be ignored by the scientific community. Just as responsible scholarly journals should not publish data from scientifically inadequate experiments, they should also not publish data from ethically inadequate experiments.

Another proposal is that such data should simply be formally destroyed.

A third proposal has been that such data not be allowable as supporting documentation for future proposed protocols. According to this proposal, ERCs would not allow the use of any such data on their application forms for ethical review of new protocols. And, according to this proposal, government agencies would also be prohibited from allowing use of any such data to support applications for drug, device, or vaccine licensure.

Serious discussion of these proposals in the biomedical ethics community could have a strengthening effect on implementation of these ethical guidelines around the world. Such a discussion would make it clear to researchers that failure to comply with these guidelines could seriously endanger the usefulness of data collected in their research.

NOTE

1. Associated Press. "Illegal AIDS testing reported." *Seattle Times* 21 September 1995, A5.

24 The Great Simple Solution

Our poor frustrated reader, now bewildered by such a large array of complex ethical quandaries, can be forgiven for desiring, and hoping to find, a Great Simple Solution. Perhaps, hopes our struggling reader, there might be found some Great Simple Solution that only the practical minded person, the person with little learning but much good sense will be able to see, the Great Simple Solution that can be seen only by a simple person of great wisdom who is able to think more clearly than all the learned people and bureaucrats put together.

I find it difficult to chastise this hope. I even share the hope myself sometimes, when my mind is overly fatigued. Three metaphors come to mind that richly express this hope: the metaphors of the egg, the knot and the empty stadium.

1 *The egg.* According to legend, Christopher Columbus once challenged all the noble men and ladies at the court dinner to see if they could balance a hard-boiled egg on the table so that it would stand upright on its small end. Everyone tried, no one succeeded. They then passed the egg back to Columbus and asked him to show them how it was done. He picked up the egg, tapped it lightly against the table on its small end to dent the shell, then set it gently and easily on the table. It stood. The problem was solved. All the learned men and ladies of the court could not solve the problem with all their trying, but Columbus, the practical man of simple wisdom, solved the problem easily.

2 *The knot.* The ancient Greek legend of the Gordian Knot tells of a great knot that was so large, so complicated, and so tightly tied that no one, not even the greatest of heroes, could untie it. Legend had it that whoever could loosen the knot would rule Asia. Great men from all over the world tried to untie the knot, but none succeeded. Finally young Alexander the Great, encountering the

problem of the great knot, simply drew his sword and cut right through the middle of the knot severing it in two. The knot was undone. It was loosened. He had provided the simple solution that none of the others had even thought of.

3 *The empty stadium.* The ancient Greek philosopher Zeno (in the fifth century BC), arguing in defense of the philosophy of Parmenides, argued that it was impossible for a man standing at one end of an empty stadium to walk across the open field to the other end of the stadium. The man could not walk across the stadium, said Zeno, because he would first have to walk half way across the stadium. But he couldn't walk even that distance because he would first have to walk half way there. But he couldn't walk even that far because he would first have to walk half way to that point. And he couldn't walk even that far because he would first have to walk half way there. And to get even that far he would first have to walk half way there. There would, of course, be an infinity of these half way points. The man would have to traverse an infinity of half way points in order to walk anywhere. No one can traverse an infinity of anything, no matter how small. Therefore, it was impossible for the man to walk anywhere, said Zeno.

Philosophers had tried for centuries to find an adequate answer to Zeno's stadium paradox. Finally one practical minded mediaeval philosopher answered thus: you solve the problem by simply standing up and walking across the stadium. That is, you quit trying to think out an answer like all the learned scholars had done. Instead, you simply stand up and walk. "It is solved by walking!" he said. "*Solvitur ambulando*," he said in Latin.

He was a practical minded man with little patience for intellectual problems and complexities. He solved the problem of how to walk across the stadium by simply standing up and walking.

Solvitur vaccinando? I can imagine our frustrated reader, or our frustrated, practical-minded activist, or even our frustrated vaccine researcher, believing that the solution to these multi-faceted ethical quandaries is to simply start doing the experiments. "Let's just start! Solvitur vaccinando," he or she might say. "It is solved by vaccinating! We are wasting our time with all this thinking and fretting. The pandemic is racing out of control. The Thesis position is correct. We must act. The problems will work themselves out as we get into the trials. We cannot afford to wait any longer!"

I have personally spoken with activists who feel this way. I have personally spoken with cooler-headed academics, even, who feel this way. Whenever and in whatever forums I have presented some of the ideas in this book, I have been able to watch members of my audience struggling to find some answer, some solution, some Great Simple Solution to all these ethical complexities. None of the proffered simple solutions, unfortunately, has yet been adequate.

Cast about as I may, I cannot see any solutions to these difficulties that are both simple and ethical. I suspect that whatever solutions we do find to these ethical complexities will not be simple ones. I suspect that any successful solutions that are developed will probably end up being just about as complex as the problems they are trying to solve.

For that reason, I am deeply encouraged and heartened when I hear WHO vaccine expert, and now director of the new Joint United Nations Programme on HIV/AIDS (UNAIDS), Dr Peter Piot, imply that every one of these ethical problems must be faced squarely and in their full complexity and must not be oversimplified, "because, with the urgent need for an effective vaccine, we cannot afford a failure due to scientific or ethical problems."[1] Failure of a trial due to scientific or design difficulties would be tragic, but even more tragic would be failure of a trial due to ethical difficulties. The discussion among ethicists of what to do with data garnered from ethically defective experiments has tended, as we saw earlier, in the direction of completely disallowing either the publication or the use of any data obtained from ethically improper research.[2] If this policy turns out to be part of the operative ethical guidelines governing the use of research data – and it may well turn out to be – then publication or use of any data from ethically defective HIV vaccine trials would be completely disallowed. The trials would have been a failure.

It is for this reason that I am encouraged to see Drs Esparza, Heyward, and Osmanov, who are leading thc WHO AIDS vaccine development efforts, as well as Dr Piot, say that the whole goal of their pretrial deliberations is to "ensure that scientifically and ethically sound Phase III HIV vaccine efficacy trials can be conducted successfully."[3]

I am heartened to hear, especially from the top, such an appreciation of the importance of the ethical.

NOTES

1. L. K. Altman MD. "After Setback, First Large AIDS Vaccine Trials Are Planned." *New York Times* 29 November 1994, B6.

   Furthermore, the international WHO panel that approved the efficacy trials referred to in the preface above also agreed with Dr Piot that no scientific or ethical shortcuts could be taken. *Ibid.*

   Another recent article reviewing the present state of vaccine trial planning, written by experts actively engaged in planning and developing those trials, also emphasizes the importance of the ethical in present trial planning. See D. F. Hoth, et al., "HIV Vaccine Development: A Progress Report," *Annals of Internal Medicine,* 8, 7, 15 October (1994) 603–11, p 609.
2. The CIOMS working group on informed consent (moderated by J. M. Last), recommended that scientific and medical journals not accept "articles based on research done without prior ethical review and without the informed and voluntary consent of the research subjects." Z. Bankowski and R. J. Levine, eds. *Ethics and Research on Human Subjects: International Guidelines (Proceedings of the XXVIth CIOMS Conference, Geneva, Switzerland, 5–7 February 1992)* (Geneva, Switzerland: Council for International Organizations of Medical Sciences (CIOMS), 1993) 228+63+x, p 57.
3. W. L. Heyward, et al., "Preparation for Phase III HIV vaccine efficacy trials: methods for the determination of HIV incidence," *AIDS,* 8, 9, September (1994) 1285–91, p 1290.

25 Thesis/Antithesis: Synthesis?

To summarize: the Thesis position, then, can be characterized as follows:

> Many of these problems will be dealt with and solved by beginning the process of designing the trials. We must initiate phase III HIV vaccine efficacy trials as soon as possible, and follow the advice of the great experimental surgeon, Dr John Hunter (professor and friend of Edward Jenner): "Don't just speculate; try the experiment."

Very little about efficacy will be learned from safety and immunogenicity trials (the numbers are too small), and less will be learned from animal experiments (since no truly adequate animal model yet exists for this disease). The only way we will learn whether these experimental vaccines will be of any actual benefit to human beings is to jump in and begin the experiments

Furthermore, we must always consider the ethics of waiting, argues the Thesis position. The increasing burden of personal tragedy, of familial and societal disruption, and of the economic and social cost associated with 10,000 new HIV infections on each day that a vaccine is not available, must also be weighed into the ethical balance.

The Antithesis position, on the other hand, can be characterized thus:

> We must do no experiments with human subjects, and especially no high-risk/low-benefit experiments, without insuring (to the fullest extent) that the rights and well-being of all individual research subjects are fully protected, as required by *The Nuremberg Code* and The CIOMS *International Ethical Guidelines for Biomedical Research Involving Human Subjects.* Otherwise we risk endangering the usefulness of data that such experiments might collect, and we also risk causing serious difficulties for biomedical researchers in the future.

That is to say, argues the Antithesis position, we must be prepared to insure:

- that prospective volunteers will have full information about all the potential harms, benefits, purposes, design, and expectations of the trial, and that their comprehension will have been appropriately assessed to insure that they do fully understand that information before they are asked for their consent to participate in the trials;
- that they are aware of what limitations there will be on researchers in protecting the confidentiality and welfare of the individual subjects;
- that their consent is free in every way, that it is uncoerced (by researchers themselves, or by anyone else in the community) and that it is free of undue inducement;
- that there is an appropriate potential-harm/potential-benefit ratio for each individual subject;
- that subjects will be protected from harm to the fullest extent possible, and/or that they will be fully compensated for any losses or harms that do befall them as a result of their participation in the trial; and
- that each prospective subject is made fully aware of their rights and responsibilities relating to their participation in the trial.

It is imperative, argues the Antithesis position, that we do not go forward with these trials until the discussions, planning, and design work have thoroughly addressed and solved all of, not just some of, these ethical problems. It is better to think things out fully before acting than to move into action without adequate thinking, and run the risk of causing more damage than can be rectified. Hundreds of thousands, perhaps millions, of lives will be directly affected by the decisions that are made surrounding these trials. We must proceed cautiously, and with great deliberation.

These are the two opposing positions. The prospect of an effective synthesis is (if Hegel can be trusted) still in the process of emergence.

26 Smallpox and Guinea Worm Disease as Metaphors

One final reflection, then a conclusion.

We have successfully eradicated only one disease from the planet, and that (smallpox) was the result of the development (extremely controversial at the time), and wise, aggressive use of a preventive vaccine. Polio may well be the third human disease to be successfully eradicated, perhaps sometime early in the next century, also by means of a preventive vaccine.

But the next disease to be eradicated from the earth, only the second one ever, will be guinea worm disease (GWD, dracunculiasis), which is expected to be gone by 1996. GWD will not be eradicated by means of a preventive vaccine, nor by means of a medication to treat sufferers from the disease, since there is no cure or very effective treatment for GWD, and people develop no immunity to it. This disease will instead be eradicated by means of changes that people make in their ways of doing things. It will be eradicated by means of individual and societal changes in behavior.

The condition commonly known as guinea worm disease, caused by the *dracunculus medinensis* parasite (the little dragon of Medina), is endemic to many parts of Africa and Asia, and has apparently, like smallpox, been causing human disease in the world since early antiquity. It seems to be as old as ancient Mesopotamia and (up until the last few years) still affected millions of people annually.

People become infected when they accidentally drink water containing a tiny crustacean which has been infected with *dracunculus* larvae. When that contaminated water reaches the person's stomach, the larvae are released; they then pass through the walls of the small intestine and take up residence in the muscles where a few of them may mature and grow to their full length, up to a meter long. They then migrate to the tissues under the armpit where the male and female eventually mate. The males soon die, but the female worm resumes her journey "just below the skin, where her outline can be seen externally, as if a bulging meter-long vein in the forearm had embarked on a subdermal voyage."

> As its maternal duties draw near, the worm navigates to its final destination: [usually to] the tissues just below the skin in a leg or foot. At this stage, the worm . . . coils and secretes a substance that produces an itching blister. The person relieves the fiery sensation by wading in water, which causes the blister to rupture. Within the crater of the ruptured blister is the reproductive opening of the female, which then sheds millions of baby worms [into the water] . . . starting the process over again.[1]

The only treatment for this painful and debilitating condition is to incise the skin and withdraw the worm. The problem is that the worm cannot simply be pulled out. The worm must be allowed to slowly let itself out of the wound, millimeter by millimeter, a process which can take a month or more. It would not do, however,

> to have a foot or two of dried worm dangling from your patients for weeks. Besides being bad advertising, dried worms catching on objects might hinder further chances of successfully removing the worm. The solution [in ancient times] was to roll up the worm on a stick. A carefully rolled worm could advertise technical know-how, something that may have been used as a symbol (viz., the caducceus) on the physician's place of practice.[2]

GWD, while not usually fatal, is still immensely debilitating, and is the direct cause of numerous person-weeks of lost labor every year in affected communities. In addition to the tragic cost to individuals in the form of pain, suffering and debilitation, GWD also takes a heavy economic toll in the villages and regions where it is endemic.

> Individual victims are often incapacitated for weeks or months by the pain and secondary infections that usually accompany emergence of the adult worms. A small fraction of victims may be crippled permanently. Many villagers are prevented from farming or attending school.

The disease also interferes with infant care, since affected mothers may be temporarily disabled.[3]

The elimination of this disease will clearly be a significant improvement in the human condition. The GWD eradication program is being coordinated by three separate organizations: Global 2000, Inc, a program of the Carter Center in Atlanta, the World Health Organization, and the US Centers for Disease Control and Prevention. Donald Hopkins,[4] who was active in the smallpox eradication program (SEP), was the first person to suggest that guinea worm disease could also be eradicated. He is now leading Global 2000's GWD eradication program (GWEP).[5]

The method by which guinea worm disease is being eliminated is a mix of the following four public health measures:

1 Educating and persuading people, in areas where the disease is endemic, to boil or filter all their drinking water every time they drink, even when away from their homes and villages. This change in behavior has actually come to pass. A very effective cloth-like filter material has even been made into hats so that it is conveniently available for filtering water at all times. Other persons can carry a small lightweight film canister with the filter cloth covering each end, so that drinking water can be poured through and filtered before consumption.
2 Sinking deep bore-hole wells for drinking water is also an important control measure since these sources of drinking water cannot be contaminated with the parasite. This measure requires persons to obtain their water from a deep well rather than from a shallow well, or from surface water.
3 Local drinking water supplies can sometimes also be treated with the chemical temephos (Abate®, made by American Cyanamid Co, Wayne, NJ) which kills the microfilaria responsible for passing the disease.
4 Public education urging infected persons to not go wading or swimming in places where drinking water is collected has also been important.

Three of these measures (1, 2, and 4) require that individual human beings change their usual behaviors. These behavioral changes, amazingly enough, have come to pass;

people have begun to boil or filter their drinking water, have sunk deep, bore-hole wells, collecting their drinking water from those wells rather than from surface waters, and they have ceased wading and swimming in areas used for drinking water. People have changed their behaviors and, as a result of these behavior changes, the disease is soon to be completely eliminated from many nations where it had been endemic for centuries. GWD is now almost completely gone from Asia,[6] and it will probably be completely eradicated from the world by 1996.

These two unequivocal public health successes, viz., smallpox eradication by means of a vaccine, and GWD eradication by means of behavior changes, may together provide a metaphor for how we will eventually (if we ever do) get some control of the spread of HIV. An HIV control program will, of course, be decisively advanced by the development and wise use of a successful preventive vaccine. Such a program will also doubtless require the implementation of significant social and individual behavior changes. There will probably need to be major changes in individual sexual behaviors, as well as major changes in societal, cultural, and religious supports for long-term, sexually-faithful partnered relationships (marriages) of both the heterosexual and homosexual variety. There will probably also need to be significant governmental changes that make for much more international communication and cooperation between governments and NGOs, particularly in matters directly relating to the public health. There will probably also need to be major social, cultural, legal, and economic reforms that provide disadvantaged and unempowered persons more control over their own well-being, and that especially will provide the world's women with much more control over matters directly and indirectly relating to their sexual lives, as well as to their status in the family and in society. And there will need to be fuller cultural and social support for the exercise of compassion toward the sick, as well as greater efforts to develop more effective antiviral drugs and treatments for opportunistic infections so that persons with AIDS and persons with HIV infection can have a better quality of life.

Such behavior changes, coupled with the wise and aggressive use of a successful preventive vaccine will probably be the only way that this epidemic will ever be satisfactorily put under control.

NOTES

1. P. Ewald. *The Evolution of Infectious Disease* (New York, NY: Oxford University Press, 1994) 298+x, p 182.
2. *Ibid.*, 182–83.
3. D. R. Hopkins, et al., "Dracunculiasis eradication: Beginning of the end," *American Journal of Tropical Medicine and Hygiene*, 49, 3 (1993) 281–89, pp 281–82.
4. See D. R. Hopkins. *Princes and Peasants: Smallpox in History* (Chicago: University of Chicago Press, 1983) 380+xx.
5. E. Bernstein. "Forward." *Medical and Health Annual, 1992.* Ed. E. Bernstein. 1992 ed. (Chicago, IL: Encyclopaedia Britannica, Inc, 1992).
6. "The most serious obstacles to eradicating dracunculiasis by 1995 are the civil war in Sudan, apathy of national and international health officials, and inadequate funding for the campaigne."E. Bernstein. "Forward." *Medical and Health Annual, 1992.* Ed. E. Bernstein. 1992 ed. Chicago, IL: Encyclopaedia Britannica, Inc, 1992). *See also* D. R. Hopkins, "Eradication of Dracunculiasis: Update," *Epidemiologic Reviews*, 13 (1991) 316–19.

27 So . . .

The Thesis position (which urges bolder action) and the Antithesis position (which urges more cautious reflection), might, despite their many disagreements, still both agree on the ultimate value of discovering a successful preventive vaccine. Both positions will probably also agree that the use of prevention measures is a much more effective way to control serious disease than the use of treatment measures. It will be better, in other words, if most people are never infected with the disease.

All the principles of human compassion do require, of course, that we make every possible effort to discover treatments for those who already suffer from the disease. But, in addition, the principles of human compassion also require that we make every possible effort to help prevent new infections in persons who are not yet infected. Preventing a disease with a vaccine, after all, eliminates the sufferings of sickness altogether, whereas a curative modality only shortens those sufferings (though this shortening is extremely valuable, of course, for those who have already contracted the disease).

The development, licensing, and aggressive use of successful vaccines for the prevention of various diseases around the world has been an enormous benefit to the public health of the world's peoples. In fact, "with the exception of safe water, no other modality, not even antibiotics, has had such a major effect on mortality reduction."[1] We can only hope that there will someday be – hopefully sooner rather than later – a vaccine that can also help diminish the incidence of HIV infection and AIDS.

If such a successful vaccine is ever discovered, tested and licensed, its successful development will be largely due to the courage, the altruism, and the heroism of the thousands, and hundreds of thousands, of individual human beings who will have volunteered for these experiments.

There will indeed be many to admire, of course – the

CEOs (Chief Executive Officers) of the pharmaceutical companies who made the difficult judgments and who undertook the great financial risks of sponsoring lengthy and expensive basic vaccine research; the directors of governmental and intergovernmental agencies (such as WHO) who have put so much effort into making these vaccine trials come to pass; the many individual researchers who took the chance of staking their careers on years-long laboratory explorations, many of which may not have paid off; ethicists and persons sitting on ethics review boards who had to make the hard choices, amidst intense passion, hope and disappointment, to approve or deny proposed research protocols; as well as many others, too numerous to mention.

But the individual persons who volunteer for these trials must not be forgotten either. They will, after all, be the ones taking the risks with their own bodies and receiving few, if any, of the benefits. Their contributions will be at least as important as the contributions of those whose names make the headlines. They too will deserve our esteem, our admiration and our lasting gratitude.

On the last page of his famous novel, *The Plague*, Albert Camus has his narrator explain to the reader that

> Dr Rieux resolved to compile this chronicle [of the plague], so that he should . . . bear witness in favor of those plague-stricken people; so that some memorial of the injustice and outrage done them might endure; and to state quite simply what we learn in time of pestilence: that there are more things to admire in men than to despise.[2]

NOTES

1. S. L. Plotkin and S. A. Plotkin. "A Short History of Vaccination." *Vaccines.* Eds. S. A. Plotkin and E. A. Mortimer, second ed. (Philadelphia, PA: W.B. Saunders Co, 1994) 1–11, p 1.
2. A. Camus. *The Plague.* Trans. Gilbert, Stuart (New York, NY: Vintage International, Random House, 1948, 1991) 308+, p 308.

Appendices

Appendix I

The Nuremberg Code (1947)

The great weight of the evidence before us is to the effect that certain types of medical experiments on human beings, when kept within reasonably well-defined bounds, conform to the ethics of the medical profession generally. The protagonists of the practice of human experimentation justify their views on the basis that such experiments yield results for the good of society that are unprocurable by other methods or means of study. All agree, however, that certain basic principles must be observed in order to satisfy moral, ethical and legal concepts:

1. The voluntary consent of the human subject is absolutely essential.

This means that the person involved should have legal capacity to give consent; should be so situated as to be able to exercise free power of choice, without the intervention of any element of force, fraud, deceit, duress, overreaching, or other ulterior form of constraint or coercion, and should have sufficient knowledge and comprehension of the elements of the subject matter involved as to enable him to make an understanding and enlightened decision. This latter element requires that before the acceptance of an affirmative decision by the experimental subject there should be made known to him the nature, duration, and purpose of the experiment; the method and means by which it is to be conducted; all inconveniences and hazards reasonably to be expected; and the effects upon his health or person which may possibly come from his participation in the experiment.

The duty and responsibility for ascertaining the quality of the consent rests upon each individual who initiates, directs or engages in the experiment. It is a personal duty and responsibility which may not be delegated to another with impunity.

2. The experiment should be such as to yield fruitful results for the good of society, unprocurable by other methods or means of study, and not random or unnecessary in nature.

3. The experiment should be so designed and based on the results of animal experimentation and a knowledge of the natural history of the disease or other problems under study that the anticipated results will justify the performance of the experiment.

4. The experiment should be so conducted as to avoid all unnecessary physical and mental suffering and injury.

5. No experiment should be conducted where there is an a priori

reason to believe that death or disabling injury will occur, except, perhaps, in those experiments where the experimental physicians also serve as subjects.

6. The degree of risk to be taken should never exceed that determined by the humanitarian importance of the problem to be solved by the experiment.

7. Proper preparations should be made and adequate facilities provided to protect the experimental subject against even remote possibilities of injury, disability, or death.

8. The experiment should be conducted only by scientifically qualified persons. The highest degree of skill and care should be required through all stages of the experiment of those who conduct or engage in the experiment.

9. During the course of the experiment the human subject should be at liberty to bring the experiment to an end if he has reached the physical or mental state where continuation of the experiment seems to him to be impossible.

10. During the course of the experiment the scientist in charge must be prepared to terminate the experiment at any stage if he has probable cause to believe, in the exercise of the good faith, superior skill, and careful judgment required of him that a continuation of the experiment is likely to result in injury, disability, or death to the experimental subject.

From *Trials of War Criminals Before the Nuremberg Military Tribunals Under Control Council Law No 10,* Vol. II. Nuremberg, Germany, October 1946–April 1949.

Appendix II

International Ethical Guidelines for Biomedical Research Involving Human Subjects

(CIOMS, WHO, Geneva, 1993)

(Basic guidelines only, without commentary)

GUIDELINE 1: INDIVIDUAL INFORMED CONSENT

For all biomedical research involving human subjects, the investigator must obtain the informed consent of the prospective subject or, in the case of an individual who is not capable of giving informed consent, the proxy consent of a properly authorized representative.

GUIDELINE 2: ESSENTIAL INFORMATION FOR PROSPECTIVE RESEARCH SUBJECTS

Before requesting an individual's consent to participate in research, the investigator must provide the individual with the following information, in language that he or she is capable of understanding:

- that each individual is invited to participate as a subject in research, and the aims and methods of the research;
- the expected duration of the subject's participation;
- the benefits that might reasonably be expected to result to the subject or to others as an outcome of the research;
- any foreseeable risks or discomfort to the subject, associated with participation in the research;
- any alternative procedures or courses of treatment that might be as advantageous to the subject as the procedure or treatment being tested;
- the extent to which confidentiality of records in which the subject is identified will be maintained;
- the extent of the investigator's responsibility, if any, to provide medical services to the subject;
- that therapy will be provided free of charge for specified types of research-related injury;
- whether the subject or the subject's family or dependants will be compensated for disability or death resulting from such injury; and
- that the individual is free to refuse to participate and will be free to withdraw from the research at any time without penalty or loss of benefits to which he or she would otherwise be entitled.

GUIDELINE 3: OBLIGATIONS OF INVESTIGATORS REGARDING INFORMED CONSENT

The investigator has a duty to:

- communicate to the prospective subject all the information necessary for adequately informed consent;
- give the prospective subject full opportunity and encouragement to ask questions;
- exclude the possibility of unjustified deception, undue influence and intimidation;
- seek consent only after the prospective subject has adequate knowledge of the relevant facts and of the consequences of participation, and has had sufficient opportunity to consider whether to participate;
- as a general rule, obtain from each prospective subject a signed form as evidence of informed consent; and
- renew the informed consent of each subject if there are material changes in the conditions or procedures of the research.

GUIDELINE 4: INDUCEMENT TO PARTICIPATE

Subjects may be paid for inconvenience and time spent, and should be reimbursed for expenses incurred, in connection with their participation in research; they may also receive free medical services. However, the payments should not be so large or the medical services so extensive as to induce prospective subjects to consent to participate in the research against their better judgment ("undue inducement"). All payments, reimbursements and medical services to be provided to research subjects should be approved by an ethical review committee.

GUIDELINE 5: RESEARCH INVOLVING CHILDREN

Before undertaking research involving children, the investigator must ensure that:

- children will not be involved in research that might equally well be carried out with adults;
- the purpose of the research is to obtain knowledge relevant to the health needs of children;
- a parent or legal guardian of each child has given proxy consent;
- the consent of each child has been obtained to the extent of the child's capabilities;
- the child's refusal to participate in research must always be respected unless according to the research protocol the child would receive therapy for which there is no medically-acceptable alternative;
- the risk presented by interventions not intended to benefit the individual child-subject is low and commensurate with the importance of the knowledge to be gained; and

- interventions that are intended to provide therapeutic benefit are likely to be at least as advantageous to the individual child-subject as any available alternative.

GUIDELINE 6: RESEARCH INVOLVING PERSONS WITH MENTAL OR BEHAVIOURAL DISORDERS

Before undertaking research involving individuals who by reason of mental or behavioural disorders are not capable of giving adequately informed consent, the investigator must ensure that:

- such persons will not be subjects of research that might equally well be carried out on persons in full possession of their mental faculties;
- the purpose of the research is to obtain knowledge relevant to the particular health needs of persons with mental or behavioural disorders;
- the consent of each subject has been obtained to the extent of that subject's capabilities, and a prospective subject's refusal to participate in non-clinical research is always respected;
- in the case of incompetent subjects, informed consent is obtained from the legal guardian or other duly authorized person;
- the degree of risk attached to interventions that are not intended to benefit the individual subject is low and commensurate with the importance of the knowledge to be gained; and
- interventions that are intended to provide therapeutic benefit are likely to be at least as advantageous to the individual subject as any alternative.

GUIDELINE 7: RESEARCH INVOLVING PRISONERS

Prisoners with serious illness or at risk of serious illness should not arbitrarily be denied access to investigational drugs, vaccines or other agents that show promise of therapeutic or preventive benefit.

GUIDELINE 8: RESEARCH INVOLVING SUBJECTS IN UNDERDEVELOPED COMMUNITIES

Before undertaking research involving subjects in underdeveloped communities, whether in developed or developing countries, the investigator must ensure that:

- persons in underdeveloped communities will not ordinarily be involved in research that could be carried out reasonably well in developed communities;
- the research is responsive to the health needs and the priorities of the community in which it is to be carried out:
- every effort will be made to secure the ethical imperative that the consent of individual subjects be informed; and

- the proposals for the research have been reviewed and approved by an ethical review committed that has among its members or consultants persons who are thoroughly familiar with the customs and traditions of the community.

GUIDELINE 9: INFORMED CONSENT IN EPIDEMIOLOGICAL STUDIES

For several types of epidemiological research individual informed consent is either impracticable or inadvisable. In such cases the ethical review committee should determine whether it is ethically acceptable to proceed without individual informed consent and whether the investigator's plans to protect the safety and respect the privacy of research subjects and to maintain the confidentiality of the data are adequate.

GUIDELINE 10: EQUITABLE DISTRIBUTION OF BURDENS AND BENEFITS

Individuals or communities to be invited to be subjects of research should be selected in such a way that the burdens and benefits of the research will be equitably distributed. Special justification is required for inviting vulnerable individuals and, if they are selected, the means of protecting their rights and welfare must be particularly strictly applied.

GUIDELINE 11: SELECTION OF PREGNANT OR NURSING (BREASTFEEDING) WOMEN AS RESEARCH SUBJECTS

Pregnant or nursing women should in no circumstances be the subjects of non-clinical research unless the research carries no more than minimal risk to the fetus or nursing infant and the object of the research is to obtain new knowledge about pregnancy or lactation. As a general rule, pregnant or nursing women should not be subjects of any clinical trials except such trials as are designed to protect or advance the health of pregnant or nursing women or fetuses or nursing infants, and for which women who are not pregnant or nursing would not be suitable subjects.

GUIDELINE 12: SAFEGUARDING CONFIDENTIALITY

The investigator must establish secure safeguards of the confidentiality of research data. Subjects should be told of the limits to the investigators' ability to safeguard confidentiality and of the anticipated consequences of breaches of confidentiality.

GUIDELINE 13: RIGHT OF SUBJECTS TO COMPENSATION

Research subjects who suffer physical injury as a result of their participation are entitled to such financial or other assistance as would compensate them equitably for any temporary or permanent impairment or disability. In the case of death, their dependants are entitled to material compensation. The right to compensation may not be waived.

GUIDELINE 14: CONSTITUTION AND RESPONSIBILITIES OF ETHICAL REVIEW COMMITTEES

All proposals to conduct research involving human subjects must be submitted for review and approval to one or more independent ethical and scientific review committees. The investigator must obtain such approval of the proposal to conduct research before the research is begun.

GUIDELINE 15: OBLIGATIONS OF SPONSORING AND HOST COUNTRIES

Externally sponsored research entails two ethical obligations:

- An external sponsoring agency should submit the research protocol to ethical and scientific review according to the standards of the country of the sponsoring agency, and the ethical standards applied should be no less exacting than they would be in the case of research carried out in that country.
- After scientific and ethical approval in the country of the sponsoring agency, the appropriate authorities of the host country, including a national or local ethical review committee or its equivalent, should satisfy themselves that the proposed research meets their own ethical requirements.

Appendix III

A Proposed Bill of Rights and Responsibilities for Participants in HIV Vaccine Trials

YOU HAVE THE RIGHT TO

- Be treated with respect by all persons connected with the research team.
- Be fully informed about:
  - the purposes, nature, and methods of the research in which you are participating;
  - all possible risks, inconveniences, hazards or discomforts of any kind related to your health or well being that might result from your participation in the trial;
  - any changes in knowledge about the vaccine being studied which could materially affect your decision to continue participation in the trial.
- Have all information relating to your participation in the trial, including whether or not you are a volunteer in the trial, and all records relating to your medical condition or serostatus, kept fully confidential and released to no one except to persons whom you explicitly, in writing, authorize to receive it.
- Be reimbursed for transportation, meals and other out of pocket expenses that result from your participation in the trial, as well as to be given a small stipend for your time involvement as described in the consent form.
- Participate in support groups, counseling sessions and classes designed for you and your family and/or partner.
- Be protected (to the fullest extent that the research team is able to protect you) from all harms, physical, psychological, social, economic and legal, which might result from your participation in these trials.
- Have the research team be on your side and looking out for your well-being.
- Be compensated for any accidental injuries which may result from your participation in the trial (as described in the consent form).
- Not be manipulated or coerced by anyone on the research team into doing anything against what you consider to be in your own best interests.
- Ask questions of the research team about anything regarding any aspect of your participation in this research project.
- Quit your participation in the trial at any time you wish, for any reason.

YOU HAVE THE RESPONSIBILITY TO

- Keep your appointments with the research team, to the best of your ability.

- Be fully truthful with the research team in your reports about risk behaviors.
- Provide fully truthful responses to counselors' questions about matters relating to your participation in the trial.
- Provide fully truthful responses on any tests or questionnaires that are part of the research.
- Keep the research team apprised of any changes in the state of your health.
- Keep the research team apprised of any changes in medications you are taking.
- Keep the research team apprised of any drugs you are taking.
- Keep the research team apprised of any changes in your residence or living situation, so they can communicate with you if they need to.
- Not "unblind" yourself, i.e., not secretly attempt to learn whether you have received the candidate vaccine or the placebo.
- Inform your counselor as soon as possible if you do inadvertently become unblinded.

____

Signature of the investigator Date

Subject's statement:

The rights and responsibilities described above have been explained to me. I have had an opportunity to ask questions. I understand that future questions I may have about my rights or responsibilities as a subject can be answered by one of the investigators.

____

Signature of subject Date

Appendix IV

Test of Understanding for Informed Consent

This is a copy of a test supplied to me from an HIV vaccine research laboratory. It was used to assess subjects' comprehension of the information they had received.

TEST OF UNDERSTANDING AND COMMITMENT [sic]

Instructions:

1. The pre-enrollment "test of understanding and commitment" is to be administered to all volunteers who meet all other inclusion and exclusion criteria for this trial, prior to signing the informed consent and being enrolled in the study. The test will be administered by protocol nurse.
2. All volunteers must answer at least 90 per cent (28 of 31) of the questions herein correctly before enrollment. The staff member administering the test may administer the test as few or as many times as necessary to allow the volunteer to successfully complete the test.

True or False Questions:

Interviewer reads to volunteer: Now, I would like to ask you some questions about your understanding of the HIV vaccine study which we have discussed with you and which you are considering joining. The purpose of these questions is to see what you know and think about this vaccine study. First I will read you a series of statements. As I read you each statement, you must tell me whether the statement is "True" or "False." Do you have any questions about what we are going to do?. . . . Can we start?

Interviewer Circles Volunteer's Response

1. AIDS is caused by a virus called HIV (Human Immuno deficiency Virus). T F
2. People who join this study will never again have to worry about catching HIV infection, no matter what they do. T F
3. Vaccines are a kind of medicine [sic] given to prevent infections. T F
4. The vaccine which is being tested in this study contains the HIV virus. T F
5. There is a very small chance that I could get HIV/AIDS from this vaccine. T F

6. This vaccine has been found to be safe for pregnant women; therefore, I may become pregnant during this study if I wish. (Women only) T F
7. If I enter this study, I may receive an inactive medication [sic] (placebo) and not the vaccine. T F
8. This study will require me to come to the vaccine center approximately 10 times during the next 8–9 months. Sometimes I may need to come in 2 days in a row. T F
9. I may develop a positive test for HIV/AIDS [sic] if I receive the vaccine, but this does not mean that I really have the virus that causes AIDS. T F
10. The vaccine could cause me to have mild fever, aches, pains and fatigue (tiredness). T F
11. This vaccine has already been proved to be effective in preventing HIV-1 infection in humans. T F
12. If I experience a serious side-effect which is judged to be due to the vaccine, I will receive care for that side-effect from medical institutions sponsoring this study. T F
13. I will be asked to give a specimen of blood only one time during this study. T F
14. People who join this study might catch HIV anyway. T F
15. People who join this study will no longer need to use condoms when they have sex with new [sic] partners. T F
16. All information about my participation in this study is strictly confidential. T F

Multiple Choice Questions: (Circle as many answers as are correct for each question.)

Interviewer reads to volunteer: For the next 3 questions, I will read a series of statements. I want you to indicate which statements are correct. Do you have any questions?

19. HIV (the virus that causes AIDS) can be transmitted in the following ways:

a. Sharing of eating utensils with someone who is already infected.
b. Having sex with someone who is already infected with HIV.
c. Sharing a needle for injecting drugs with someone who is already infected with HIV.
d. Hugging someone who is already infected with HIV.
e. Receiving a blood transfusion from a person who is infected with HIV.
f. From a mother infected with HIV to her unborn baby.

20. Potential side-effects of participating in this study include:

a. Soreness in the arm at the site of injection for a day or two after the injection.
b. Minor bleeding or bruising at the site where blood is taken from arm.
c. The possibility of getting HIV/AIDS from this vaccine.
d. A brief period of lightheadedness or faint feeling after having blood drawn.
e. A positive blood test for HIV/AIDS [sic].

21. Which of the following are true statements about this vaccine study?

a. This vaccine may provide protection from HIV/AIDS, so therefore, I should not be concerned with avoiding high risk behavior such as having sex with prostitutes or multiple partners.
b. My participation will require approximately 10 visits to the vaccine center during working hours. Some visits will be short, requiring less than 1 hour; however, some visits may require 2 or 3 hours of my time away from work, school or family.
c. I will be compensated for my time away from work, transportation to the vaccine center and meal expenses which result from my participation.
d. The vaccine being used in this study has been approved to be tested in humans by the FDA in Thailand and the United States.

Interviewer to volunteer: Thank you for taking this test with me. I would now like to go over the questions and your answers with you. This will be a chance for you to ask any questions you may still have about HIV/AIDS or this vaccine study.

Test of Understanding and Commitment [sic]

Phase I Safety and Immunogenicity Trial of [a candidate peptide vaccine].

Answer Key:

1. T
2. F
3. T
4. F
5. F
6. F
7. T
8. T
9. T
10. T
11. F
12. T
13. F
14. T
15. F
16. T

19.
a. Incorrect
b. Correct
c. Correct
d. Incorrect
e. Correct
f. Correct

20.
a. Correct
b. Correct
c. Incorrect
d. Correct
e. Correct

21.
a. Incorrect
b. Correct
c. Correct
d. Correct

Appendix V

Proposed Application Forms for Ethical Review

Form for detailing potential harms to subjects

(Complete one form for each potential harm to subjects and society in the study. Attach these forms to the Form for requesting ethical review of HIV vaccine trial.)

I. **Type of candidate vaccine**

II. **The potential harm:** ______________________________

to individual	☐	physical	☐
to society	☐	psycho-social	☐
		economic	☐

III. **Estimated seriousness of the suffering**

miniscule ☐
mild ☐
moderate ☐
serious ☐
severe ☐
comments:

IV. **Estimated percent likelihood that this harm will occur**

extremely unlikely ☐
not likely ☐
fairly likely ☐
very likely ☐
completely unknown ☐

Reasons for this estimate:

V. **When is this harm likely to occur in a volunteer's life?**

VI. **What steps will you take to minimize the chances of this harm occurring?**

VII. **What remedies will you offer if this harm does occur?**

VIII. **What compensations will you make available to volunteers if the harm occurs?**

IX. **Assessing understanding**

A. What method will you use to inform prospective volunteers of the nature, severity and likelihood of this harm?

B. What method will you use to assess whether each prospective volunteer has understood the nature, severity and likelihood of this harm?

Form to Request Ethical Review of HIV Vaccines

I. **Type of vaccine**
II. **Research sponsor**

Principal investigator
Funding source

III. Preliminary research

A. Laboratory research performed

Summary of results

B. Animal research

Summary of results

C. Phase I human trials

Summary of results

D. Phase II human trials

Summary of results

IV. Potential harms

A. To individual volunteers

i. Potential physical harms
(List each harm separately, and include the following)
a. Nature of harm
b. Estimated seriousness of suffering
miniscule ☐
mild ☐
moderate ☐
serious ☐
severe ☐
comments:

c. Estimated degree of likelihood that it will occur
extremely unlikely ☐
not likely ☐
fairly likely ☐
very likely ☐
completely unknown ☐
1) Reasons for this estimate
d. When the harm might occur in volunteer's life
e. Steps sponsors will take to prevent this harm
f. Remedies if this harm does occur
g. Compensation to volunteer if the harm occurs

ii. Potential psycho-social harms
(List each harm separately, and include the following)
a. Nature of harm
b. Estimated seriousness of suffering
miniscule ☐
mild ☐
moderate ☐
serious ☐
severe ☐
comments:

c. Estimated degree of likelihood that it will occur

extremely unlikely ☐
not likely ☐
fairly likely ☐
very likely ☐
completely unknown ☐

1) Reasons for this estimate

d. When the harm might occur in volunteer's life
e. Steps sponsors will take to prevent this harm
f. Remedies if this harm does occur
g. Compensation to volunteer if the harm occurs

iii. Potential economic harms
(List each harm separately, and include the following)
a. Nature of harm
b. Estimated seriousness of suffering

miniscule ☐
mild ☐
moderate ☐
serious ☐
severe ☐
comments:

c. Estimated degree of likelihood that it will occur

extremely unlikely ☐
not likely ☐
fairly likely ☐
very likely ☐
completely unknown ☐

1) Reasons for this estimate

d. When the harm might occur in volunteer's life
e. Steps sponsors will take to prevent this harm
f. Remedies if this harm does occur
g. Compensation to volunteer if the harm occurs

B. To society

i. Potential physical harms
(List each harm separately, and include the following)
a. Nature of harm
b. Estimated seriousness of suffering

miniscule ☐
mild ☐
moderate ☐
serious ☐
severe ☐
comments:

c. Estimated degree of likelihood that it will occur

extremely unlikely ☐
not likely ☐
fairly likely ☐
very likely ☐
completely unknown ☐

1) Reasons for this estimate

d. When the harm might occur in society

e. Steps sponsors will take to prevent this harm

f. Remedies if this harm does occur

g. Compensation to society if the harm occurs

ii. Potential psycho-social harms

(List each harm separately, and include the following)

a. Nature of harm

b. Estimated seriousness of suffering

miniscule ☐
mild ☐
moderate ☐
serious ☐
severe ☐
comments:

c. Estimated degree of likelihood that it will occur

extremely unlikely ☐
not likely ☐
fairly likely ☐
very likely ☐
completely unknown ☐

1) Reasons for this estimate

d. When the harm might occur in society

e. Steps sponsors will take to prevent this harm

f. Remedies if this harm does occur

g. Compensation to society if the harm occurs

iii. Potential economic harms

(List each harm separately, and include the following)

a. Nature of harm

b. Estimated seriousness of suffering

miniscule ☐
mild ☐
moderate ☐
serious ☐
severe ☐
comments:

c. Estimated degree of likelihood that it will occur

extremely unlikely ☐
not likely ☐
fairly likely ☐
very likely ☐
completely unknown ☐

1) Reasons for this estimate

d. When the harm might occur in society

e. Steps sponsors will take to prevent this harm

f. Remedies if this harm does occur

g. Compensation to society if the harm occurs

V. Potential benefits

A. To individual volunteers

i. Potential physical benefits
(List each benefit separately, and include the following)
a. Nature of benefit
b. Estimated importance of benefit
not very important ☐
moderately important ☐
very important ☐
comments:
c. Estimated degree of likelihood that it will occur
extremely unlikely ☐
not likely ☐
fairly likely ☐
very likely ☐
completely unknown ☐
1) Reasons for this estimate
d. When this benefit might occur in the volunteer's life
1) Reasons for this estimate

ii. Potential psycho-social benefits
(List each benefit separately, and include the following)
a. Nature of benefit
b. Estimated importance of benefit
not very important ☐
moderately important ☐
very important ☐
comments:
c. Estimated degree of likelihood that it will occur
extremely unlikely ☐
not likely ☐
fairly likely ☐
very likely ☐
completely unknown ☐
1) Reasons for this estimate
d. When this benefit might occur in the volunteer's life
1) Reasons for this estimate

iii. Potential **economic** benefits
(List each benefit separately, and include the following)
a. Nature of benefit
b. Estimated importance of benefit
not very important ☐
moderately important ☐
very important ☐
comments:
c. Estimated degree of likelihood that it will occur
extremely unlikely ☐
not likely ☐

fairly likely ☐
very likely ☐
completely unknown ☐
1) Reasons for this estimate
d. When this benefit might occur in the volunteer's life
1) Reasons for this estimate

B. To society

i. Potential physical benefits
(List each benefit separately, and include the following)
a. Nature of benefit
b. Estimated importance of benefit
not very important ☐
moderately important ☐
very important ☐
comments:
c. Estimated degree of likelihood that it will occur
extremely unlikely ☐
not likely ☐
fairly likely ☐
very likely ☐
completely unknown ☐
1) Reasons for this estimate
d. When this benefit might occur in society
1) Reasons for this estimate

ii. Potential psycho-social benefits
(List each benefit separately, and include the following)
a. Nature of benefit
b. Estimated importance of benefit
not very important ☐
moderately important ☐
very important ☐
comments:
c. Estimated degree of likelihood that it will occur
extremely unlikely ☐
not likely ☐
fairly likely ☐
very likely ☐
completely unknown ☐
1) Reasons for this estimate
d. When this benefit might occur in society
1) Reasons for this estimate

iii. Potential economic benefits
(List each benefit separately, and include the following)
a. Nature of benefit
b. Estimated importance of benefit
not very important ☐
moderately important ☐

very important ☐
comments:

c. Estimated degree of likelihood that it will occur
   - extremely unlikely ☐
   - not likely ☐
   - fairly likely ☐
   - very likely ☐
   - completely unknown ☐

   1) Reasons for this estimate

d. When this benefit might occur in society
   1) Reasons for this estimate

VI. Motivations to volunteer

(List each possible motivation separately)

A. The motivation: ______________________________

B. Is this motivation likely to be satisfied or not?
   - extremely unlikely ☐
   - not likely ☐
   - fairly likely ☐
   - very likely ☐
   - completely unknown ☐

C. Reasons for this estimate

VII. Informed consent

Include a copy of the study's informed consent form.

VIII. Assessing comprehension

A. List the elements in the above sections which you consider important for prospective volunteers to know about

B. List the methods you will use to inform prospective volunteers of those elements

C. List the methods you will use to assess whether each of these elements has been understood by the prospective volunteers before asking for their consent

Selected Bibliography

The Belmont Report: Ethical Principles and Guidelines for the Protection of Human Subjects of Research. National Commission for the Protection of Human Subjects of Biomedical and Behavioral Research, Department of Health, Education and Welfare, 1979.

G. L. Ada, "Modern Vaccines," *The Lancet,* 335, 3 March (1990) 523–26.

L. K. Altman MD. "After Setback, First Large AIDS Vaccine Trials Are Planned." *New York Times* 29 November 1994, B6.

G. J. Annas and M. A. Grodin, eds. *The Nazi Doctors and the Nuremberg Code: Human Rights in Human Experimentation* (New York, NY: Oxford University Press, 1992) 371+xxii.

Associated Press. "Gambian group have rare immunity to AIDS virus." *The Seattle Times* 1 January 1995.

Associated Press. "Illegal AIDS testing reported." *Seattle Times* 21 September 1995, A5.

Associated Press. "Researchers Look to Girl, 13, for Clues on AIDS." *The New York Times* 9 January 1995. A10.

M. Balter, "UN Readies New Global AIDS Plan," *Science,* 266.25 November (1994) 1312–13.

Z. Bankowski, ed. *International Guiding Principles for Biomedical Research Involving Animals* (Geneva, Switzerland: Council for International Organizations of Medical Sciences (CIOMS), 1985) 28.

Z. Bankowski, ed. *International Guidelines for Ethical Review of Epidemiological Studies* (Geneva: World Health Organization, 1991).

Z. Bankowski. *International Ethical Guidelines for Biomedical Research Involving Human Subjects* (Geneva, Switzerland: Council for International Organizations of Medical Sciences (CIOMS), 1993) 63.

Z. Bankowski and R. J. Levine, eds. *Ethics and Research on Human Subjects: International Guidelines (Proceedings of the XXVIth CIOMS Conference, Geneva, Switzerland, 5–7 February 1992)* (Geneva, Switzerland: Council for International Organizations of Medical Sciences (CIOMS), 1993) 228+63+x.

S. Barnet, et al., "An AIDS-like Condition Induced in Baboons by HIV-2," *Science,* 266, No 5185, October 28 (1994) 642.

R. Bayer. "Confidentiality and Its Limits." *Ethics and Law in the Study of AIDS.* Eds. H. Fuenzalida-Puelma, A. M. L. Parada and D. S. LaVertu. (Washington, DC: Pan American Health Organization, Regional Office of the World Health Organization, 1992) Scientific Publication No. 530: 145–47.

T. L. Beauchamp and J. F. Childress. *Principles of Biomedical Ethics.* Third ed. (New York: Oxford University Press, 1989) 470+x.

R. B. Belshe, et al., "Interpreting HIV Serodiagnostic Test Results in the 1990s: Social Risks of HIV Vaccine Studies in Uninfected Volunteers," *Annals of Internal Medicine,* 121, 8, 15 October (1994) 584–89.

R. Berkow and A. J. Fletcher, eds. *The Merck Manual of Diagnosis and Therapy*. Fifteenth ed. (Rahway, NJ: Merck Sharp & Dohme Research Laboratories, 1987) 2697+xxviii.

E. Bernstein. "Forward." *Medical and Health Annual, 1992*. Ed. E. Bernstein. 1992 ed. Medical and Health Annual (Chicago, IL: Encyclopaedia Britannica, Inc, 1992).

G. Bjune and T. W. Gedde-Dahl, "Some problems related to risk-benefit assessments in clinical testing of new vaccines," *IRB*, 15, 1, January–February (1993) 1–5.

E. Blackstone, personal communication about UW's vaccine research studies, 22 July 1994.

D. Blum. *The Monkey Wars* (New York, NY: Oxford University Press, 1994) 306+xii.

T. Brown and P. Xenos. "AIDS: Epidemic in Asia." *Seattle Post-Intelligencer* 2 October 1994, D1, D3.

D. S. Burke, "Human HIV Vaccine Trials: Does antibody-dependent enhancement pose a genuine risk?," *Perspectives in Biology and Medicine*, 35, 4, Summer (1992) 511–30.

C. Burrell for the Associated Press. "Report: 'Reckless' use of Gulf War drugs." *Seattle Times* 8 December 1994, A3.

D. Butler, "Call for International AIDS policy," *Nature*, 372, 24 November (1994) 308.

M. Caldwell, "The Long Shot," *Discover*, August (1993) 61–69.

A. Camus. *The Plague*. Trans. Gilbert, Stuart (New York, NY: Vintage International, Random House, 1948, 1991) 308+.

N. A. Christakis, "The Ethical Design of an AIDS Vaccine Trial in Africa," *Hastings Center Report*, 18, 3, June/July (1988) 31–37.

J. Cohen, "At Conference, Hope for Success Is Further Attenuated," *Science*, 266, 18 November (1994) 1154.

J. Cohen, "Bumps on the Vaccine Road," *Science*, 265, 2 September (1994) 1371–73.

J. Cohen, "The Duesberg Phenomenon," *Science*, 266.9 December (1994) 1642–49.

S. S. Connor. "International Legal and Ethical Aspects of Developing and Distributing an HIV Vaccine." *Ethics and Law in the Study of AIDS*. Eds. H. Fuenzalida-Puelma, A. M. L. Parada and D. S. LaVertu. (Washington, DC: Pan American Health Organization, Regional Office of the World Health Organization, 1992) 162–69.

P. Cotton, "International Disunity on Vaccine Efficacy Trials," *JAMA*, 272, Number 14, 12 October (1994) 1090–91.

G. Cowley and M. Hager. "The Ever-Expanding Plague." *Newsweek*, 22 August 1994: 37.

J. Crewdson. "AIDS Vaccine Fails Researcher." *Chicago Tribune* Sunday 5 September 1993, 1.

A. W. Crosby. *America's Forgotten Pandemic: The Influenza of 1918* (New York City, NY: Cambridge University Press, 1989) 337+xiv.

M. Daniel, et al., "Protective effects of a live attenuated SIV vaccine with a deletion in the nef gene," *Science*, 258 (1992) 1938–41.

K. M. De Cock MD, MRCP, DTM&H, et al., "The Public Health Implications of AIDS Research in Africa," *JAMA*, 272, 6, 10 August (1994) 481–86.

P. Duesberg. *Inventing the AIDS Virus* (Washington, DC: Regnery, 1996) 722.

G. Eddy, personal communication about HIV vaccine, 4 July 1994.

Editor, "Editorial," *Nature*, 366, 6455, 9 December (1993) 493–94.

Editor, *The Bulletin of the King County Medical Society*, 73, 12, December (1994) cover.

S. Efron. "Russia moves toward AIDS tests for foreigners." *Seattle Times* 29 October 1994, A3.

P. Ewald. *The Evolution of Infectious Disease* (Oxford University Press, 1994).

P. Ewald, personal communication about virulence, 15 July 1994.

K. Fackelmann, "HIV's infectious nature," *Science News*, 14 January (1995) 22.

D. FitzSimons, personal communication, 1994.

D. P. Francis. "A Private-Sector AIDS Vaccine? Don't Hold Your Breath." *Washington Post* 19 July 1994, A17.

M. B. Gardner and S.-L. Hu, "SIV vaccines, 1991 – a year in review," *AIDS*, 5 (supplement 2) (1991) S115–S127.

L. Garrett. *The Coming Plague: Newly Emerging Diseases in a World Out of Balance* (New York, NY: Farrar, Straus and Giroux, 1994) 750+xiv.

L. Garrett. "Unified AIDS Fight; UN combines agency efforts." *Newsday* 13 December 1994, A37.

Global Programme on AIDS. *Statement from the Consultation on Criteria for International Testing of Candidate HIV Vaccines* (Geneva: World Health Organization, 1989) 13.

Global Programme on AIDS. *Potential for WHO-Industry Collaboration on Drug and Vaccine Development for HIV/AIDS* (Geneva: World Health Organization, 1993) 11.

M. F. Goldsmith, "For AIDS Treatment, Vaccines, Now Think Genes," *JAMA*, 269, 17, 5 May (1993) 2189–90.

C. Grady RN, PhD. *The Search for an AIDS Vaccine* (Indianapolis, IN: Indiana University Press, 1995) 193.

M. D. Grmek MD, PhD. *History of AIDS: Emergence and Origin of a Modern Pandemic.* Trans. Maulitz, Russell, and Duffin, Jacalyn (Princeton, NJ: Princeton University Press, 1990) 279+xii.

B. F. Haynes, "Scientific and Social Issues of Human Immunodeficiency Virus Vaccine Development," *Science*, 260, 28 May (1993) 1279–86.

D. A. Henderson and F. Fenner. "Smallpox and Vaccinia." *Vaccines*. Ed. S. A. Plotkin. Second ed. (Philadelphia, PA: W.B. Saunders Company, 1994) 13–40.

W. L. Heyward, et al., "Preparation for Phase III HIV vaccine efficacy trials: methods for the determination of HIV incidence," *AIDS*, 8, 9, September (1994) 1285–91.

D. Hodel and AIDS Action Foundation Working Group. *HIV Preventive Vaccines: Social, Ethical, and Political Considerations* (AIDS Action Foundation, Office of AIDS Research, National Institutes of Health, 1994).

J. Homsy et al., "The Fe and Not CD4 Receptor Mediates Antibody Enhancement of HIV Infection in Human Cells," *Science*, 244 (1989) 1357–59.

D. R. Hopkins. *Princes and Peasants: Smallpox in History* (Chicago: University of Chicago Press, 1983) 380+xx.

D. R. Hopkins, et al., "Dracunculiasis eradication: Beginning of the end," *American Journal of Tropical Medicine and Hygiene,* 49 3 (1993) 281–89.

D. F. Hoth, et al., "HIV Vaccine Development: A Progress Report," *Annals of Internal Medicine,* 8, 7, 15 October (1994) 603–11.

A. R. Jonsen, "The Ethics of Using Human Volunteers for High-Risk Research," *Journal of Infectious Diseases,* 160, August (1989) 205–208.

A. R. Jonsen and J. Stryker, eds. *The Social Impact of AIDS in the United States* (Washington, DC: National Academy Press, 1993) 322+xiv.

I. Kant. *Fundamental Principles of the Metaphysic of Morals.* Trans. Thomas Kingsmill Abbott, vol 42 of 54, (Chicago, IL: The Great Books of the Western World, Encyclopedia Britannica, Inc, 1785, 1952).

E. Kessel, "Estimating Risks and Benefits in AIDS Vaccine and Drug Trials," *AIDS & Public Policy Journal,* 5, 4, Winter (1990) 186–88.

S. Kierkegaard, *Concluding Unscientific Postscript.* Trans. D. Swenson and W. Lowrie (Princeton University Press, 1846, 1941) 577+xxii.

J. Kinsella. *Covering the Plague: AIDS and the American Media* (New Brunswick, NJ: Rutgers University Press, 1989) 299+x.

Knight-Ridder-Newspapers. "AIDS extremely contagious in early stages, study finds." *The Seattle Times* 6 January 1995, A7.

W. C. Koff, "Development and Testing of AIDS Vaccines," *Science,* 241 (1988) 426–32.

W. C. Koff, "The Next Steps Toward a Global AIDS Vaccine," *Science,* 266, 25 November (1994) 1335–37.

M. Lappé. *Evolutionary Medicine: Rethinking the Origins of Disease* (San Francisco, CA: Sierra Club Books, 1994) 255+xii.

A. J. Levine. *Viruses* (New York, NY: Scientific American Library, 1992) 241+xii.

C. Levine, N. N. Dubler and R. J. Levine, "Building a New Consensus: Ethical Principles and Policies for Clinical Research on HIV/AIDS," *IRB,* 13, 1–2, January–April (1991), 1–17.

R. J. Levine. *Ethics and Regulation of Clinical Research.* Second ed. (New Haven, CT: Yale University Press, 1986, 1988) 452+xx.

R. J. Levine. "AIDS Research and Ethical Review Boards." *Ethics and Law in the Study of AIDS.* Eds. H. Fuenzalida-Puelma, A. M. L. Parada and D. S. LaVertu. (Washington, DC: Pan American Health Organization, Regional Office of the World Health Organization, 1992) 170–77.

A. Mack, ed. *In Time of Plague: The History and Social Consequences of Lethal Epidemic Disease* (New York: New York University Press, 1991) 206+xii.

J. Mann and D. Tarantola. *AIDS in the World: Redefining the Global HIV/AIDS Pandemic* (New York: Oxford University Press, in press).

J. Mann, D. Tarantola and T. Netter, eds. *AIDS in the World* (Cambridge, MA: Harvard University Press, 1992) 1037+xvi.

E. Martin. *Flexible Bodies: Tracking Immunity in American Culture, from the Days of Polio to the Age of AIDS* (Boston: Beacon Press, 1994) 320+xxiv.

J. R. Mascola MD, J. G. McNeil MD, MPH and D. S. Burke MD, "AIDS Vaccines: Are We Ready for Human Efficacy Trials?," *Journal of the American Medical Association,* 272, 6, August 10 (1994) 488–89.

M. J. McElrath and L. Corey. "Current Status of Vaccines for HIV." *Pediatric AIDS: The challenge of HIV infection in infants, children and adolescents.* Eds. P. H. Pizzo and C. M. Wilfert (Baltimore, MD: Williams and Wilkins, 1994) 869–887.

W. H. McNeill. *Plagues and Peoples* (Garden City, NY: Doubleday Anchor, 1976) 340+xii.

J. Miller, "Ethical Standards for Human Subject Research in Developing Countries," *IRB, A Review of Human Subjects Research,* 14.3, May–June (1992) 7–8.

P. Monette. *Borrowed Time* (New York, NY: Avon, 1988) 342.

E. Mozes-Kor. "The Mengele Twins and Human Experimentation: A Personal Account." *The Nazi Doctors and the Nuremberg Code: Human Rights in Human Experimentation.* Eds. G. J. Annas and M. A. Grodin. (New York, NY: Oxford University Press, 1992) 53–59.

National Public Radio. *Program on Vaccines,* 1994.

R. O'Boyle. *Living With AIDS* (Seattle, WA: The Seattle Times, 1992) 62.

J. W. Pape et. al., "The Urge for an AIDS Vaccine: Perspectives from a Developing Country," *AIDS Research and Human Retroviruses,* 8, 8 (1992) 1535–37.

B. Peabody. *The Screaming Room* (New York, NY: Avon, 1986) 279.

J. C. Petricciani, W. C. Koff and G. L. Ada, "Efficacy Trials for HIV/AIDS Vaccines," *AIDS Research and Human Retroviruses,* 8, 8 (1992) 1527–29.

P. Piot Associate Director of WHO's GPA. *Lecture on Global Issues for HIV Prevention and Control.* Harborview Medical Center: University of Washington, 13 July 1994.

S. A. Plotkin MD and E. A. Mortimer Jr, MD, eds. *Vaccines.* Second ed. (Philadelphia: W.B. Saunders Company, 1994) 996+xix.

S. L. Plotkin and S. A. Plotkin. "A Short History of Vaccination." *Vaccines.* Eds. S. A. Plotkin and E. A. Mortimer. Second ed. (Philadelphia, PA: W.B. Saunders Co, 1994) 1–11.

J. P. Porter, M. J. Glass and W. C. Koff, "Ethical Considerations in AIDS Vaccine Testing," *IRB, A Review of Human Subjects Research,* 11, 3, May–June (1989) 1–4.

E. D. Prentice, et al., "Bill of Rights for Research Subjects," *IRB, A Review of Human Subjects Research,* 15, 2, March–April (1993) 7–9.

N. R. Rabinovich, et al., "Vaccine Technologies: View to the Future," *Science,* 265, 2 September (1994) 1401–04.

C. A. Radin. "AIDS fight portrayed as a failure; Prevention, education efforts fall short, global specialist says." *The Boston Globe* 10 August 1994, 1.

A. J. H. Rains MS, FRCS. *Edward Jenner and Vaccination. Pioneers of Science and Discovery* (East Sussex: Wayland Publishers, 1974, 1980) 96.

Reuters. "WHO Approves Large-Scale AIDS Vaccine Trials." *Centers for Disease Control AIDS Daily Update* 14 October 1994.

A. Richardson and D. Bolle, eds. *Wise Before Their Time: People from Around the World Living with AIDS and HIV Tell Their Stories* (London: Harper Collins, 1992) 144.

W. N. Rida and D. N. Lawrence, "Some Statistical Issues in HIV Vaccine Trials," *Statistics in Medicine,* 13 (1994) 2155–77.

I. Roitt. *Essential Immunology*. Seventh ed. (Oxford: Blackwell Scientific Publications, 1991) 356+xii.

R. Root-Bernstein. *Rethinking AIDS: The Tragic Cost of Premature Consensus* (New York, NY: The Free Press, Macmillan, 1993) 512+xv.

D. J. Rothman. *Strangers at the Bedside: A history of how law and bioethics transformed medical decision making* (Basic Books, HarperCollins, 1991) 303+xii.

S. Rowland-Jones, "HIV-specific Cytotoxic T-cells in HIV-exposed but Uninfected Gambian Women," *Nature Medicine*, 1 January (1995) 59–64.

F. Ryan MD. *The Forgotten Plague: How the Battle Against Tuberculosis was Won – and Lost* (published in England as *The Greatest Story Never Told*). (Boston: Little, Brown and Co, 1992, 1993) 460+xx.

B. D. Schoub. *AIDS & HIV in Perspective* (New York, NY: Cambridge University Press, 1994) 268+xx.

C. Siebert. "Smallpox is Dead, Long Live Smallpox." *The New York Times Magazine* 21 August 1994, section 6, 31–55.

L. M. Simons. "AIDS cure impossible this century, predicts co-discoverer of virus." *The Seattle Times* 8 August 1994.

S. Sontag. *AIDS and Its Metaphors* (New York: Farrar, Straus and Giroux, 1988) 95.

W. P. &. S. T. Staff. "Radiation tests involved at least 23,000." *Seattle Times* 22 October 1994, A1.

J. R. Starke and K. K. Connelly. "Bacille Calmette-Guérin Vaccine." *Vaccines*. Eds. S. A. Plotkin MD and E. A. Mortimer Jr, MD. Second ed. (Philadelphia: W.B. Saunders Company, 1994) 439–73.

P. Stehr-green, personal communication about vaccines, 4 January 1995

G. Stine. *Acquired Immune Deficiency Syndrome: Biological, Medical, Social and Legal Issues*. First ed. (Englewood Cliffs, NJ 07632: Prentice Hall, 1993) 462+xxxii.

S. Stolberg. "Promise, Disappointment Mark AIDS Vaccine Quest." *Los Angeles Times* 9 August 1994, A1.

L. Thomas. *The Fragile Species* (New York, NY: Charles Scribner's Sons, 1992) 193+xii.

L. Thompson. "CDC Reorganization Prompts Concern," *Science*, 266, 25 November (1994) 1313.

Thucydides. *The History of the Peloponnesian War*. Vol. 6 of *Great Books of the Western World*. Trans. Crawley, Richard, and Feetham, R. 6 of 54, (Chicago: Encyclopedia Britannica, 1952) 267.

M. ul Haq, ed. *Human Development Report 1994*. (New York, NY: Oxford University Press, 1994) 226+xii.

UNDP. *Human Development Report 1994* (United Nations Development Programme, 1994).

B. G. Weniger. "Experience from HIV incidence cohorts in Thailand: implications for HIV vaccine efficacy trials," *AIDS*, 8, 7 (1994) 1007–1010.

WHO. *Malaria vaccine reduces disease in African children*. World Health Organization, 28 October 1994.

E. B. Wilson. *At the Edge of Life: an introduction to viruses*. NIH Publication 80–433 (Washington DC: US Department of Health and Human Services, Government Printing Office, 1980) 75.

Index